Update in Infectious Diseases

Edited By

Viroj Wiwanitkit

Wiwanitkit House, Bangkhae, Bangkok Thailand 10160

CONTENTS

i

PREFACE

Infectious disease is an important group of medical disorder. This is still a public health problem for all countries around the world. It is still the leading course of death. There are many epidemics of new emerging and remerging infectious diseases at present and this warrants the necessity to update our knowledge on infectious diseases. Fighting up with infectious diseases, collaboration between health care workers and non health care workers is required. The construction of the knowledge exchange *via* the E-book series can be useful. The series of E-book on this area can be the integrated source of knowledge among the experts and workers on several facets of infectious diseases. This is the first volume of the series containing the articles relating to the situation in Thailand, a country with a center of excellence for tropical medicine.

Viroj Wiwanitkit
Wiwanitkit House
Bangkok
Thailand

CONTRIBUTORS

Viroj Wiwanitkit	Professor, Wiwanitkit House, Bangkhae, Bangkok Thailand; Professor of Tropical Medicine, Visiting Professor, Hainan Medical College, Hainan, China
Nutchya Khemnak	Physician, Faculty of Medicine, Chulalongkorn University, Bangkok, Thailand
Saranya Namrassamiwong	Physician, Faculty of Medicine, Chulalongkorn University, Bangkok, Thailand
Jamsai Suwansaksri	Associate Professor, Faculty of Allied Health Science, Chulalongkorn University, Bangkok, Thailand
Paungpen Chunhapran	Associate Professor, Faculty of Nursing, Naresuan University, Phitsanulok, Thailand
Akkaradej Suyaphan	Administrator, Mae Jam Hospital, Chiangmai, Thailand
Kunakorn Atchaneeyasakul	Physician, Faculty of Medicine, Chulalongkorn University, Bangkok, Thailand
Pongsathorn Kue-a-pai	Physician, Faculty of Medicine, Siriraj Hospital, Mahidol University, Bangkok, Thailand

CHAPTER 1

A STORY ON EMERGING AND ENDEMIC NEUROLOGICAL INFECTION IN THAIALND

Viroj Wiwanitkit[1]

[1]Wiwanitkit House, Bangkhae, Bangkok Thailand 10160

Address correspondence to: Professor Viroj Wiwanitkit, Wiwanitkit House, Bangkhae, Bangkok Thailand 10160 Email: wviroj@yahoo.com

Abstract: Neurological infection seems to be an important group of infectious disease. This group of disorders has become an important focus in neurology and general medicine. In Thailand, there are many interesting emerging and endemic neurological infections. In this specific chapter, the author will present details of some interesting clinical reports on important emerging and endemic neurological infection in Thailand.

Keywords: Neurological, infection.

1. INTRODUCTION

Neurological infection seems to be an important group of infectious disease. This group of this disorder becomes an important focus in neurology and general medicine. In Thailand, there are many interesting emerging and endemic neurological infections. Due to the nature of neurological infection, the described infection is usually fatal and needs proper management.

In this specific chapter, the author will present details of some interesting clinical reports on important emerging and endemic neurological infection in Thailand.

2. GRANULOMATOUS AMOEBIC ENCEPHALITIS IN THAILAND

Introduction

Granulomatous amoebic encephalitis (GAE) is a very rare disease of the brain [1]. *Acanthamoeba* spp., is the principal protozoa that is commonly referred to as pathogenic free-living amoeba causing GAE [2-3]. GAE occurs very rarely but it occurrence usully relates to high fatality. Until present, fewer than 150 cases of GAE have been identified and noted worldwide [1-3]. *Acanthamoeba* spp. are ubiquitouse free-living amoeba that can be found in a very wide range of environmental settings including in soil, water and air [2-5]. *Acanthamoeba* spp. are highly resistant to disinfectants, temperature variation and desiccation and this protozoa is also responsible for the serious infection in human beings, GAE. Basically, GAE is often associated with patients with acquired immunodeficiency status [6]. In GAE, there are, most likely, common foci of the pathogenic protozoa in lungs and skin and the rearching to the terminal, the CNS, is usually owing to the hematogenous spreading process [7]. Luckily, GAE is not a disease transmitted from person to person [1-4].

In Thailand, the first case report of GAE has been published since Jariya by *et al.* [8]. Since the first case report, there have been sporadic case reports of the GAE in Thailand. Here, the author performed a literature review on the reports of GAE in Thailand in order to study the clinical summary of the GAE among the Thai patients.

Materials and Methods

This study was designed as a descriptive retrospective study. A literature review on the papers concerning GAE in Thailand was performed. The author hereby performed the standard literature review on GAE reports in Thailand from database of the published workds cited in the Index Medicus and Science Citation Index. The author also reviewed the published works in all 256 local Thai journals, which is not included in the international citation index, for the report of GAE in Thailand. The literature review was focused on the period 1992 to 2009. According to the literature review, there are 5 reports meeting the criteria and all 5 reprots were recruited for further study. The details of clinical presentation of the patients (such as clinical manifestation, history of risk behavior, length of stay in the hospital, diagnosis, treatment and discharge status) in all included reports were studied in depth. The demographic data of all cases including age , sex and address were reviewed as well. Descriptive statistics were used in analyzing the patients' characteristics and laboratory parameters for each group. All the statistical analyses in this study were made using SPSS 7.0 for Windows Program.

Results

Due to this study, there have been at least reports of 11 GAE, of which 3 cases were non lethal (Table 1). The mean age was 40.8 + 22.4 years (range 17 years-82 years) with male: female ratio equaled to 5: 6. According to our series, 7 cases (63.6 %) had underlying diseases causing impaired immunity (Table 1). Concerning the left 4 cases without underlying immunocompromised status, only 1 cases (9.1 %) had history of exposure to water. The patients's clinical features on the admission are shown in Table 2. impairment of consciousness, high fever, headache and stiff neck are the four main common clinical features. On admission, complete blood count (data available in 9 cases) showed average white blood count equaled to 7.8 ± 4.3 x 1000 WBC/mm^3 (range = 2.1-16.6 WBC/mm^3) with average relative neutrophil count equal to 69.1 ± 18.8 % (rabge 38-90 %). The lumbar puncture (data available in 6 cases revealed increased whie blood count (average = 244.2 ± 367.9 WBC/mm^3; range = 9-940 WBC/mm^3) with mononuclear cell predominance (average = 75.5 ± 32.9 %; range = 20-100 WBC/mm^3). Average CSF protein and glucose were 488.5 ± 486.3 mg/dL and 50.9 ± 28.8 mg/dL (range = 18-92 mg/dL), respectively.

In three cases, the primary diagnoses of GAE were made by detection of the organism in the cerebrospinal fluid (CSF). The other cases were primarilty diagnosed by autopsy. All death cases died within 2 weeks after admission (average = 5.6 ± 2.5 weeks, range 1.5-2 months). Of all death cases, autopsy studied were performed and revealed the brain pathology as diffuse necrotic vasculitis with several Acanthamoeba trophozoites and cysts, diffuse hemorrhagic encephalomalacia and diffuse granulomas.

Discussion

GAE is the most deadly infection of the central nervous system apart from rabies. It is rare but fatal. Until present, less than 150 cases have been noted worldwide, from the United State, England, Eastern Europe, Africa and Asia [1-4]. However, the causative organism is thermophilic and grows well in tropical and subtropical climates, therefore, most cases have been noted from the mentioned area [1-4]. In Thailand, the GAE is sporadically noted since 1992 [6]. In this review, only 11 Thais with GAE were detected and used for further analysis [8-12]. The clinical symptoms and signs that are found in our GAE summarized cases were similar to those in the previous report [13]. The symptoms and sign as impairment of consciousness, fever, headache and stiff neck can be found in all cases. According to these findings, most cases of GAE are usually misdiagnosed as meningitis and delayed for treatment. In this study, the subjects are from several age groups. Most had underlying immunodeficiency disorder. Different from Naegeria infection [1-2], the subjects had rarely previous history of water exposure. In addition, the period of onset is longer.

Concerning the laboratory investigation, the neutrophilia can be detected from complete blood count. While in most cases, the CSF profile presented the mononuclear pleomorphic. Nevertheless, the detection of amoebic trophozoite in the CSF is rare. Indeed, detection of organism in the CSF required experience microscopist. According to our series, in almost all cases, organisms cannot be detected in the CSF despite there were numerous organisms detected from autopsy study. Therefore, these items can be another cause of delayed specific treatment. In our series, some cases had already treated as the bacterial infection before. Concerning the cases, which organisms could be detected from CSF examinations, early definitive diagnosis and good outcome of treatment can be yielded [10].

Table 1. Clinical presentations of the 11 Thai cases of GAE.

No	Year (authors)	Age (years)	Sex	Add-ress*	Period of onset	Length of Hospitali-zation	Primary Diagnosis	Underlyin g disease	Treatment	Final status
1	1992 (Jariya *et al.*)	50	Female	NE	N/A	N/A	Autopsy	No	No specific treatment	Dead
2	1994 (Sangruchi *et al.*)	26	Female	N/A	N/A	N/A	Autopsy	SLE	No specific treatment	Dead
3	1994 (Sangruchi *et al.*)	20	Female	N/A	N/A	N/A	Autopsy	Chronic ulcer	No specific treatment	Dead
4	1994 (Sangruchi *et al.*)	20	Male	N/A	N/A	N/A	Autopsy	Aplastic	No specific treatment	Dead
5	1994 (Sangruchi *et al.*)	48	Female	N/A	5 days	N/A	Autopsy	Anemia	No specific treatment	Cure
6	1998 (Nidanandana *et al.*)	64	Male	C	1 day	30 days	CSF examination	Chronic	Rifampicin, Amphotericin B	Cure
7	1998 (Nidanandana *et al.*)	82	Male	C	14 days	63 days	CSF examination	Alcoholism	Rifampicin, Amphotericin B	Cure
8	1998 (Nidanandana *et al.*)	62	Female	C	5 days	30 days	CSF examination	Steroid misusage	Rifampicin, Amphotericin B	Dead
9	2000 (Arayawichainont *et al.*)	43	Male	N/A	30 days	42 days	Autopsy	Alcoholic cirrhosis	Ampicillin, cefotaxime	Dead
10	2000 (Arayawichainont *et al.*)	17	Male	N/A	6 days	21 days	Autopsy	SLE	Anti TB, Bactrim	Dead
11	2001 (Wanachiwanawin)	17	C	42 days	56 days	Autopsy	No	No	Rifampicin, Amphotericin B ketoconazole	Dead

* address is classified according to the Region of Thailand; NE = Northeastern, C = Central

** N/A means not noted in the literature

Table 2. Clinical manifestations on admission in 11 cases with GAE.

Clinical manifestations	Numbers of patients (%)
Impaired of consciousness	9
Headache	8
Fever	8
Stiff neck	7
Convulsion	4
Weakness	4

Concerning the treatment and outcome, our study also agrees that GAE is really fatal disease. However, there are three non-fatal cases in our series [10]. These three cases were early diagnosed. Concerning these cases, the combination of intravenous amphotericin B and oral rifampicin for 1-2 months cure the patient with no recurrence [10]. Two of the three cured cases had complete recovery while the other one had permanent neurodeficit as sequelae. These three cases are ones of non-fatal GAE, a very rare condition, of which the total records less than 10 in the literature [1-4]. In conclusion, the GAE is a fatal CNS infection, which is sporadically noted in Thailand but it remains a public health importance. The clinical diagnosis of GAE is usually difficult because of the sparsely of cases and unfamiliarity with the infections of clinicians. The prognosis outcome is usually grave. The recommended treatment regimen is amphotericin B and rifampicin.

Conclusion

Granulomatous amoebic encephalitis (GAE) is a very rare but deadly infection of the central nervous system. Until present, fewer than 150 cases have been observed and noted worldwide. Here, the author performed a literature review on the reports of GAE in Thailand in order to study the clinical summary of GAE among the Thai patients. This study was designed as a descriptive retrospective study. A literature review of the papers concerning GAE in Thailand was performed. Due to this study, there have been at least reports of 11 GAE, of which 3 cases were non-lethal. The mean age was 40.8 + 22.4 years with male: female ratio about 5: 6. Underlying immunocompromised status can be demonstrated in 7 cases. Concerning the patients' clinical features, impairment of consciousness, high fever, headache and stiff neck are the four main common clinical characteristics. The subjects are from different age groups and from many provinces in various regions of Thailand. Concerning the laboratory investigation, the CSF profile presented the lymphocytic pleomorphic. Trophozoite could be identified in only three cases in this series and these three cases are non-fatal. In conclusion, GAE is sporadically noted in Thailand but it remains a public health issue. The clinical diagnosis of GAE is usually difficult because many clinicians are unfamiliar with the disease. The prognosis outcome is usually grave. The recommended treatment regimen is amphotericin B and rifampicin.

3. PSEUDALLESHCHELIA BOYDII BRAIN ABSCESS, SOME NOTES FROM THE LATEST CASE FROM THAILAND

Generally, systemic scedosporiasis due to the anamorph or asexual form *Pseudallescheria boydii* (*Scedosporium apiospermum*) has become an important cause of opportunistic mycosis, especially in patients undergoing high-risk hematopoietic stem cell transplantation [14]. It can be mistaken, histologically, for *Aspergillus* Spp. Howecer, *P. boydii* is clinically distinguished by resistance to most antifungals and its ability to cause invasive mycoses in immunocompetent patients. There are at least 26 noted cases of *P. boydii* brain abscesses from 1965 to 2004 with only four survivors. The last case is in Thailand: a famous singer got this infection, still in the hospital, and becomes a well-known topic for the general population as well as the most famous infected case [15].

From the literatures, there are two groups of patients, a) the immunocompromised subjects, especially for those who got transplantation and b) the immunocompetent subjects with the history of near drowning. Most cases usually developed CNS symptoms gradually as the nature of CNS fungal infection [16-17]. The recent widely used antifungal, which mentioned for effective therapeutic effect, is voriconazole [16]. Due to the widely practiced transplantation and the dirty contaminated water in the city drainage at the present day, the risk of getting this infection might be higher than the past. The awareness of this infection, which can lead to early diagnosis and prompt treatment, is necessary.

4. NEUROCYSTICERCOSIS, MANIFESTATIONS AND NEUROPATHOLOGY IN THAI CASE REPORTS

Taeniasis is a parasitic disease that is caused by the ingestion of contaminated raw pork or meat. The main clinical manifestation for all taeniasis is the intestinal taeniasis. Considering intestinal taeniasis, most of the cases are asymptomatic. The most common complaint is passage (active or passive) of proglottids, which is associated with slight discomfort. Other symptoms include colicky abdominal pain (more common in children), nausea and diarrhea. For *T. solium*, the neurocysticerosis is another important clinical manifestation. Concerning the neurological involvement of *T. solium*, cysticercosis, infection occurs following oral ingestion of eggs of the porcine tapeworm, *T. solium* [18].

This study was designed as a descriptive retrospective study. A literature review on the case reports of neurocysticercosis in Thailand was performed. The author performed the literature review from database of the published works cited in the Index Medicus and Science Citation Index. The author also reviewed the published works in all 256 local Thai journals, which is not included in the international citation index, for the report of neurocysticercosis in Thailand. The clinical presentation as well as the outcome in all included reports were summarized.

In this work, 19 repors [19-37] covering 127 Thai cases of neurocysticercosis were derived for further analysis. In this series, the initial presentation was as seizure disorder (120 cases, 94.5 %), raised intracranial tension (86 cases, 67.7 %), meningoencephalitis (17 cases, 13.4 %), psychiatric manifestation (3 cases, 2.4 %) and parkinsonism (1 case, 0.8 %). Some cases had more than one clinical presentation. The lesions can be detected at cerebrum in 112 cases, cerebellum in 12 cases, cerebellopontine in 1 case, pontomedulla in 1 case, ventricle in 1 case and foramen monro in 1 case. There is a case with combined infection of intracerebral sparganosis. Age incidence was ranged from 6 years to 74 years, male to female ratio was 2: 1. The diagnosis by radiological findings of calcified cysts or nodules can be seen in 121 cases (95.3 %). There is only 6 fatal cases (4.7 %) in this study and all of the death cases had the diagnosis by autopsy. In 27 documented cases, abnormalities in cerebrospinal fluid were mild pleocytosis and mild elevation of protein.

Concerning the treatment, medical and surgical treatments were used in 84 cases and 37 cases respectively. For those who received medical treatment, albendazole and praziquantel was used in 52 cases and 32 cases, respectively. After treatment, the results can be divided into two patterns; (a) the lesions were disappeared completely (97 cases) and (b) improved with sequelae (24 cases). There is no difference in the outcome from the different treatments.

5. REFERENCES

1.   Martinez AJ. Free-living amphizoic and opportunistic amebas. Brain Pathol 1997; 7: 583-983.

2.   Parija SC, JAkakeethee SR. Negleria lowleri: a free living amoeba of emerging medical importance. J Commun Dis 1999; 31: 153-9.

3.   Walker CW. Acnathamoeba: ecology, pathogenicity and laboratory detection. Br J Biomed Sci 1996; 33: 146-51.

4.   Ockert G. Review article: occurrence, parasitism and pathogenicity potency of free-living ameba. Appl Parasiol 1993; 34: 77-88.

5.   Rodriguez-Zaragoza S. Ecology of free-living amoebas. Crit Rev Microbiol 1994; 20: 225-41.

6.   Ferrante A. Free-living amoeba: pathogenicity and immunity. Parasite Immunol 1991; 13: 31-47.

7.   Scaglia M. Scaglia M. Human pathology caused by free-living amoeba. Ann Ist Super Sanita 1997; 33: 551-66.

8.   Jariya P, Lertlaituan P, Warachoon K. Acanthamoeba spp: a cause of chronic granulomatous amoebic encephalitits. Siriraj Hosp Gaz 1992; 44: 148-53.

9.   Sangruchi T, Martinex AJ. Visvesvara GS. Spontaneous granulomatous amebic encephalitis: report of four cases from Thailand. Southeast Asian J Trop Med Public Health 1994; 25: 309-13.

10.   Nidanandana S, Leelayoova S. Report of three patients of Acanthamoeba meningoencephalitis and literature review. Royal Thai Army Med J 1998; 51: 235-9.

11.   Arayawichainont A, Chawalparit O, Sangruchi T, Senanarong V. Granulomatous amebic encephalitis: report of two patients with neyroimaging finding. Asian J Radiol 2000; 5: 83-9.

12.   Wanachiwanawin D. What have we learnt from recent infection of the pathogenic free-living protozoa in Thailand. Presented at the Joint International Tropical Medicine Meeting 2001. Bangkok Thailand 8 -10 August, 2001

13.   Lu D, Luo X, Xu Q, Li C. A clinico-pathological study of granulomatous ameobic encephalitis. Zhonghua Bing Li Xue Za Zhi 1999; 28: 169-73.

14. Safdar A, Papadopoulos EB, Young JW. Breakthrough Scedosporium apiospermum (Pseudallescheria boydii) brain abscess during therapy for invasive pulmonary aspergillosis following high-risk allogeneic hematopoietic stem cell transplantation. Scedosporiasis and recent advances in antifungal therapy. Transpl Infect Dis 2002; 4: 212-7.

15. Injured Thai pop star taken off respirator, moved from intensive care. Utusan (2003, December 9) Available at Http: // http: //health.surfwax.com/files/Abscesses.html.

16. Nesky MA, McDougal EC, Peacock Jr JE. Pseudallescheria boydii brain abscess successfully treated with voriconazole and surgical drainage: case report and literature review of central nervous system pseudallescheriasis.

17. Hachimi-Idrissi S, Willemsen M, Desprechins B, Naessens A, Goossens A, De Meirleir L, Ramet J. Pseudallescheria boydii and brain abscesses. Pediatr Infect Dis J 1990; 9: 737-41

18. Bales HW. Neurocysticercosis: migration of a parasite. J Am Acad Nurse Pract. 2000; 12: 240-8.

19. Nunrungroj W, Charoenhirunyingyos S, Chisevikul R, Wanachiwanawin D, Eamsobhana P, Mahakittikun V. Neurocysticercosis: clinical manifestations and assessments. Siriraj Hosp Gaz 2002; 54: 394-402.

20. Nakchang Y, Jenjittranunt C. A 30 years old female patients with history of seizure and pain at both legs. Clinic 1999; 15: 239-240.

21. Chotmongkol V. Cerebral cysticercosis : clinical manifestation and the result of treatment with praziquantel within 2 years. Srinagarind Hosp Med J 1990; 5: 1-9.

22. Techathuvanan S. Cysticercosis : 5-year review at Rajavithi Hospital. J Rajavithi Hosp 1998; 8: 33-41.

23. Tantajumroon T, Thitasut P. Cysticercosis with report of 3 cases of cysticercosis cerebralis. J Med Assoc Thai 1964; 49: 515-528.

24. Pothawananont S. The treatment of intraparenchymal cerebral cysticercosis by Albendazole : a case report. Reg 6 Med J 1992; 6: 371-378.

25. Punyanitya S. The treatment of intraparenchymal cerebral cysticercosis by albendazole: a case report. Bull Dept Med Serv 1991; 16: 253-255.

26. Kasemsant D, Navacharoen N, Kangsanarak J, Laowong M. Cerebellopontine angle cysticercosis : a case report. J Otolaryngol Head Neck Surg 1994; 9: 37-43.

27. Anutrakoolchai K. Neurocysticercosis: case report. Saraburi Hosp Med J 1996; 21: 27-30.

28. Sujittranit L. Brain cysticercosis in pediatric patients at Maharaj, Chiangmai. Thai J Pediatr 1996; 35: 40.

29. Chotmongkol V. Albendazole for neurocysticercosis. Srinagarind Hosp Med J 1991; 6: 93-99.

30. Tansanee P. Neurocysticercosis presenting with Parkinsonism : a case report. Bull Dept Med Serv 1992; 17: 565-569.

31. Sangcham K, Handagoon P. Cerebral cysticercosis presenting as a mass lesion obstructing the ventricular system. Bull Dept Med Serv 1987; 12: 433-438.

32. Chulamok I. CNS cysticercosis. R Thai Army Med J 1996; 39: 431.

33. Pongprasert S. Foramen monro cysticircus cyst. Bull Lampang Hosp 1986; 7: 19-28.

34. Punyadasaniya V. Cysticercosis of the nervous system. R Thai Army Med J 1972; 25: 437-455.

35. Leelachaikul P, Chuahirun S. Cysticercosis of the thyroid gland in severe cerebral cysticercosis : report of a case J Med Assoc Thai 1978; 60: 405-410.

36. Tangchai P. Clinico-pathological-conference. Chula Med J 1968; 13: 89-99.

37. Pongprasert S. Sparganum mansoni combined with cysticercus cellulosae infected in pontomedullary junction in the same patient, presented with two clinical states : a case report. Bull Lampang Hosp 1985; 6: 225-250.

CHAPTER 2

PREVALENCE OF INTESTINAL PARASITE AND SELF-PREVENTION BEHAVIORS OF VILLAGERS IN A RURAL VILLAGE AFTER OPISTHORCHIS VIVERRINI CONTROL PROGRAM, MAHASARAKAM, PROVINCE THAILAND**

Viroj Wiwanitkit[1], Puangpen Chunhapran[2] and Jamsai Suwansaksri[3]

[1]*Wiwanitkit House, Bangkhae, Bangkok Thailand 10160;*

[2] *Faculty of Nursing, Naresuan University, Phitsanulok;*

[3] *Department of Clinical Chemistry, Faculty of Allied Health Sciences, Chulalongkorn University, Bangkok 10330 Thailand*

** Presented at the Joint International Tropical Medicine Meeting 2001. Bangkok Thailand August 8-10, 2001

Address correspondence to: Professor Viroj Wiwanitkit, Wiwanitkit House, Bangkhae, Bangkok Thailand 10160 Email: wviroj@yahoo.com

Abstract: *Opisthorchis viverrini* is an important trematode infection in the Northeastern Region of Thailand.Following a number of epidemiology studies and trial projects, the national liver fluke control program has been developed and operated under different National Public Health Development Plans. Presently, the program is being operated and focused on the northeastern provinces of Thailand. A survey in Non Sam Ran village, Borabue District, Mahasarakam Province where the high prevalence of opisthorchiasis was mentioned, was performed during October 1999. The setting was a village under the control program with annual praziquantel distribution. A brief survey of self-prevention behaviors towards intestinal parasite infection of the villagers was performed. Purposive sampling of 56 villagers from each available house in the village was performed. According to the questionnaires, all villagers admitted wearing shoes, avoiding eating raw food and using toilet. However, some (44.6 %) still disclosed using hand without washing before eating. In interest, most (89.3 %) replied self-prescribing antihelminthic drug to get rid of their own intestinal parasites. Furthermore, we also performed stool examination in all 56 sampled villagers (16.2 %). In interest, there was no case of opisthorchiasis. However, 7 cases (12.5 %) of Ascaris lumbricoides infection and 7 cases (12.5 %) of Entamoeba spp infection were detected. Comparing to other nearby setting without previous control program, low prevalence of trematode infection in our studied community is detected. However, the high prevalence of nematode and protozoa infections in this setting was still observed. Nevertheless, some poor hygienic practice such as using hands without washing before eating, due to the traditional belief are still detected.

Keywords: *Opisthorchis viverrini*, infection, control program.

1.INTRODUCTION

Among pathogenic parasitic infections in the Northeastern Region of Thailand, liver fluke infection is one of the highest prevalence [1]. This disease has been prevalent in this area for more than 4 decades [2]. Therefore, the control program of opisthorchiasis in this region was set by the Department of Communicable Disease Control (CDC), Ministry of Public Health Thailand since 1984.

The program focused on the community level by performing yearly stool screening test and distribution of anti-fluke drug, praziquantel, as well as health education. As a result, the reduction in the prevalent rate of opisthorchiasis can be observed. The prevalence of the disease decreased from 34.6 % in 1984 to 18.5 % in 1994 [2]. However, a large variation of infected rate (5.20-56.25 %) was observed [2]. This means that there might be some pitfalls of the program in some specific areas. Therefore, a field study to study the effectiveness of the program in each setting is necessary [1].

Here, we report our field study in a rural area of Mahasarakham Province of the Northeastern Region of Thailand. This area is under the control program with annual distribution of praziquantel. In interest, we detected low prevalence of trematode infection in our studied community compared to the nearby setting without previous control program. However, the high prevalence of round worm and protozoa infections in this setting was still observed. Nevertheless, some poor hygienic practice such as using hand without washing before eating, due to the traditional belief are still detected.

2. MATERIALS AND METHODS

Study area and participants

The setting of this survey was at Non Sam Ran village, Borabue District, Mahasarakam Province. Its location is about 450 km from Bangkok, capital of Thailand. The study area is the endemic area of liver fluke infections under the fluke control program. The previous prevalence of the trematode infection in this area before implementation of fluke control program was about 45 %(noted by the community hospital, Borabue hospital).

The fluke control program has been operated mainly by the community hospital, focusing on improving food and environmental sanitation towards trematode infection and annual distribution of praziquantel. This control program has been introduced to this village for years but there is no report of the prevalence of trematode infection in this community after the control program. Therefore, we performed this study as a pilot study.

This survey was performed during 23-28 October, 1999. In cooperation of local health workers, and community leaders who assisted us in maximizing community participation and compliance. The people in this area were willing to participate in the study. Verbal informed consent was obtained from each individual before the study.

Questionnaire survey

A brief survey of self-prevention behavior towards intestinal parasite infections of the villagers was performed. Purposive sampling of 56 villagers (16.2 % of total villagers) from all available households in the village was performed. The questionnaire focused on the important preventive habits towards parasitic infections such as wearing shoes, eating habit, toilet habit and self-prescription.

Stool examinations

All 56 sampled villagers (16.2 % of total villagers) were also recruited into the field laboratory study. A label carton was distributed to each subject for stool collection. All subjects were explained for the importance of stool examination and asked for verbal informed consent. Stool specimens were obtained from all participants and examined for the presence of intestinal parasite eggs or larvae as previously described [5-6]. About ten grams of each stool specimen were collected. Stool examination was performed microscopically using a direct smear technique at the camp by the medical technologists.

Data analysis

All data were statistically analyzed by the Microsoft Excel 6.0 programs. Comparison of our results to the results of a recent previous study [6] in the nearby setting without previous control program was also performed. The difference between relative frequencies of parasitic infection was tested by proportional Z test [7].

3. RESULTS

Characteristics of study population

Cartons were provided to 56 residents in Non Sam Ran village, Borabue District, Mahasarakam Province, at the time of our visit. All individuals returned their stool samples the next day. Of the 56 individuals examined for intestinal parasites, 26 were males and 30 were females.

Questionnaire survey

According to the questionnaire survey, all villages replied wearing shoes, avoiding eating raw food and using toilet. However, some (44.6 %) still replied using hand without washing before eating. In interest, most (89.3 %) replied self-prescribing antihelminthic drug to get rid of their own intestinal parasites (Table 1).

Parasitism in the studied population

From stool examination in 56 villagers, intestinal parasites were recovered in 14 individuals (Table 2), giving the infection rate was 25 %. In interest, there was no case of opisthorchiasis. However, 7 cases (12.5 %) of Ascaris lumbricoides infection and 7 cases (12.5 %) of Entamoeba spp infection were detected.

Comparing to the result of the recent previous study in the nearby village without control program, a statistical significant lower relative frequency of fluke infection was observed (P < 0.05) (Table 3).

Table 1. Practice according to the preventive habits.

Practice	Number (%) of subject who replied	
	Yes	No
1. Using toilet include hand-washing with soap after toileting	56 (100 %)	0 (0 %)
2. Using hand without washing before eating	25 (44.6 %)	31 (55.4 %)
3. eating raw food	56 (100 %)	0 (0 %)
4. self-prescribing antihelminthic drug	50 (89.3 %)	6 (10.7 %)

Table 2. Relative prevalence of parasitism.

Parasites	Total number of subjects/ Infected subject	
	Male	Female
	(n = 26)	(n = 30)
Ascaris lumbricoides	3	4
Entamoeba coli	3	4
Opisthorchis viverrini	0	0

Table 3.   Relative frequencies of intestinal parasite infection in our study and the recent previous study in a nearby setting without fluke control program.

Intestinal parasite infection	Relative frequencies of intestinal parasite infection (%)		P value
	Present study	Previous study*	
(n = 56)	(n = 153)		
With any parasite infection	25	92	P < 0.05
With Trematode infection	0	89	P < 0.05

* previous study in a nearby setting without fluke control program (Wiwanitkit *et al.*, 2001 [6])

4. DISCUSSION

Parasitic infections affect more than 35 % of the Thai population [8]. In the past, the data showed that the highest prevalence of helminthic infections in the Northeastern Thailand was due to the liver fluke, Opisthorchis viverrrini [2, 9]. During 1953 and 1981, the shooting of prevalence of the liver fluke infection from 25 % to 34.6 % of the population was observed [2]. Therefore, the

Department of communicable Disease Control (CDC) of the Thai Ministry of Public Health has been established the national liver fluke control program. Many centers of fluke control unit were set such as in Khon Kaen and Roi Et. Subsequently, control on a region -wide scale was included in the sixth 5 -year National Public Health Development Plan (1987-1991). As a result, the decrease in the prevalence of the disease to 11.8 % in 1996 was observed [1].

Here we noted the pilot survey result in Non Sam Ran village, Borabue District, Mahasarakam Province where the high prevalence of trematode infection was mentioned. After the long-term trematode control program, our study showed that the null prevalence of trematode infection. However, due the nature of pilot study, the sample size appears too small to comment on the lack of prevalence of the liver fluke. However, comparing to the previous prevalence before the control program (45 %), a significant lower can be observed. Nevertheless, this study could match a recent study of Triteeraprapab *et al.* [5], which also mentioned the low prevalence in the nearby area under the same control program.

Although ours showed a very low prevalence of opisthorchaisis a high prevalence of ascariasis can be detected. Also this result is similar to that of Triteeraprapab *et al.* [5], which mentioned the high prevalence of hookworm after the liver fluke control program. A possible explanation may relate to the annual distribution of the praziquantel, the effective drug for opisthorchiasis. Because the first drug of choice for both hookworm and Ascaris lumbricoides is not the praziquantel, therefore, poor effectiveness in getting rid of these two parasites can be expected.

Furthermore, from our brief questionnaires, although the villagers presented some satisfied practice such as avoiding eating raw food and using toilet in disposal of excreta, poor hygienic practice can be detected. In interest, 44.6 % of the surveyed subjects still replies using hand without washing before eating. All gave the reason according to their traditional lifestyle. Also they mentioned that this eating method could provide good taste. Therefore, it may be another possible explanation for some intestinal parasite infection in this village.

Another interesting malpractice detected in our study was the self-prescribing antihelminthic drug, praziquantel, to get rid of their own intestinal parasites. This practice can be harmful because of overdose and side effects of the antihelminthic drug. Health education about this topic is necessary. We also raised the problem that how much the poor hygienic practice like this is in the other communities.

However, some limitation of this study must be mentioned. This study is only a pilot study with small sample size therefore generalization of the results to the other setting must be carefully considered. Consequently, one cannot extrapolate this to mean that praziquantil administration has controlled the parasitic infection. Second, the method used for stool examination in this study is not the concentration technique due to the limitation of the field study. However, a recent previous report mentioned the acceptable result of using the simple smear as a screening tool [6]. Finally, due to the Thai traditional, adult Thai people do not like to let anybody sees their stools, therefore, it is difficult to get a large amount of stool sample. To cope with this problem, our teams tried our best attempt to explain the villagers, use label carton to avoid lost and exchange of stool sample and perform home visit in this study. Although there are some limitation due to the nature of this study, nevertheless, this study can be a good case study for this topic.

Besides the liver fluke control program, environmental interventions, were as necessary to other soil-helminthes and that eating habit is still the big problem according to the high prevalence of intestinal parasitic infection among the population in the Northeastern Thailand. Health education and control of other non fluke parasites should also be accompanied with the fluke control program. Furthermore, to strengthen the national program, planning, monitoring and supervision for all operational elements have to be seriously considered [2].

5. ACKNOWLEDEGEMENT

We are thankful to all of the villagers who participated into this study. We also would like to thank Professor Schelp FP, who give very useful advice and review of our work.

6. REFERENCES

1.   Jongsuksantigul P. Control of helminth infections of Thailand. Tropical Infectious disease: Now and Then. Presented at the Medical Congress in Commemoration of the 50th Anniversary of the Faculty of Medicine, Chulalongkorn University; Jun 3-6, Bangkok Thailand Bangkok: Faculty of Medicine, Chulalongkorn University, 1997.

2.   Jongsuksantikul P, Imsomboon T. The impact of a decade long opisthorchiasis control program in northeastern Thailand. Southeast Asian J Trop Med Public Health. 1997; 28: 551-7.

3.   Triteeraprapab S, Akrabovorn P, Promtorng J, Chuenta K. High prevalence of hookworn infection in a population of Northeastern Thailand after an opisthorchiasis control program. Chula Med J 1999; 43: 99-108.

4.   Triteeraprapab S, Jongwutiwses S, Chanthachum N, The prevalence rates of human intestinal parasites in Mae-la-moong. Umphang District, Tak Province , a rural area of Thailand. Chula Med J 1997; 41: 649-58.

5.   Triteeraprapab S, Nuchprayoon I, Eosinophilia, anemia, and parasitism in a rural region of Northwest Thailand. Southeast Asian J Trop Med Public Health 1998; 29: 584-90.

6.   Wiwanitkit V, Suwansaksri J, Nithiuthai S. Prevalence of intestinal parasite among the local people in a village without previous history of antihelminthic drug distribution, Lum Pra Due village, Nakhonratchasrima, Thailand. Presented at the Joint International Meeting on Tropical Medicine 2001; Aug8- 10, Bangkok Thailand, 2001.

7.   Walpole RE, Myers RH. Probability and Statistics of Engineering and Scientists. New York: McMillan, 1972.

8.   Communicalbel Disease Division. Report: National Survey of Parasitic Infections. Bangkok: Communicable Disease Division, CDC Department, Ministry of Public Health 1996.

9.   Jongsuksantikul P, Chaeychomsri W, Techamontrikul P. Study on prevalence and intensity of intestinal helminthiasis and opisthorchiasis in Thailand. J Trop Med Parasitol 1992; 15 : 80-95.

CHAPTER 3

PARASITIC CONTAMINATION IN WATER AND SOIL: A BRIEF REVIEW

Viroj Wiwanitkit[1]

[1]*Wiwanitkit House, Bangkhae, Bangkok Thailand 10160*

Address correspondence to: Professor Viroj Wiwanitkit, Wiwanitkit House, Bangkhae, Bangkok Thailand 10160 Email: wviroj@yahoo.com

Abstract: An important problem at present is the contamination of drinking water. In this paper, the author will focus on the parasitic contamination in water and further implication on human health. The important parasites that are usually mentioned as major contaminants will be briefly reviewed. In addition to water contamination, soil contamination is another important problem. Basically, soil contamination with pathogenic parasite is a big public health problem in tropical developing countries. Diseases transmitted by soil are common in many tropical areas, including Thailand. In this article, the author summarized the prevalence of soil contamination with pathogenic parasite in Thailand. According to analysis, overall prevalence of contamination is equal to 7.8 %. There is no significant correlation between setting and prevalence.

Keywords: contamination, parasite, water, soil.

1. WATER CONTAMINATION BY PARASITE

Introduction

Water is important for all human beings. Drinking water is necessary for maintenance of life. An important problem at present is the contamination of drinking water. Indeed, there are several kinds of contamination such as toxic substance contamination and microbial contamination. In this paper, the author will focus on the parasitic contamination in water and further implication on human health. The important parasites that are usually mentioned as major contaminants will be briefly reviewed.

Crytosporidium spp contamination in water

Cryptosporidium species are protozoan parasites that are increasingly recognized as an important and widespread parasite causing enteric disease in humans and other animals [1]. The severity of infection can vary mainly depending on the species and the immune status of the host. Whilst there are several species of Cryptosporidium which have the potential to infect humans, the most important are *C. hominis* (which is largely a human infection) and *C. parvum* (which is a zoonotic infection). Cryptosporidiosis tends to be self-limiting in the immunocompetent host, but is particularly serious for immunocompromised patients because there is no curative method for the disease [2]. Cryptosporidia are transmitted via the fecal-oral route primarily by consumption of contaminated foods or water. Many epidemics were associated to foodstuffs and the potential for contamination with the transmissive stages of Cryptosporidium parvum is gaining increasing attention [3-7]. Coasts and rivers can be contaminated by the presence of Cryptosporidium oocysts, if these water environments are polluted by anthropogenic and livestock fecal discharges [8-9].

The direct threat of contaminated water to human is not much because most contaminated water samples are not normal drinking water but water in river or canal. However, the problem usually occurs due to further contamination in bivalve shellfish in the seashore where the contaminated water is collected. Basically, most marine bivalve shellfish feed on suspended phytoplankton, which are trapped from water pumped across the gills by ciliary action [10]. Melo *et al.* [10] said that pathogenic microorganisms in the water may be filtered by the gills during feeding, and become concentrated in the digestive glands/tract hence it could expect that marine bivalve shellfish could act as transmission vehicles for outbreaks of protozoan infections in humans. Therefore, the presence of Cryptosporidium oocysts in sea food is an important public health concern. At present, survey of Cryptosporidium oocysts in sea food should be set up in endemic areas. Concerning the techniques for determination, the two main techniques are immunological and molecular biological methods.

For example, Miller *et al.* [11] studied clams (*Corbicula fluminea*) as bioindicators of fecal contamination with Cryptosporidium spp. in freshwater ecosystem. According to this work, Miller *et al.* noted that oocyst dose and clam collection time were significant predictors for detecting oocysts in shellfishes [11]. Gómez-Couso *et al.* [12] determined the levels of detection of Cryptosporidium oocysts in shellfishes and noted a 31.1% of contamination and only one species, *C. parvum*. In another study of Gomez-Bautista *et al.* [13], infective C. parvum oocysts were detected in shellfishes from a shellfish-producing region and reached the conclusion that sea animals especially shellfish were important reservoir hosts of C. parvum infection for humans.

Giardia spp contamination in water

Giardia are water-borne parasites that cause gastroenteritis in humans and can potentially shorten the life spans of immunocompromised individuals [14]. The transmissive stages are their cysts which are resistant to environmental stresses and water treatment practices [14]. Although Giardia spp. are commonly noted as enteric protozoa in several countries, their real transmission to human via drinking water remains unclear. In southeast Asia, investigations on the contamination of water supplies with Giardia are very few data has previously described on the parasite cyst detection in water environment [15-16]. *Giardia* spp contamination in drinking water is very important and becomes public health concern. Kent *et al.* [17] proposed that the risk of giardiasis associated with unfiltered surface water systems. LeChevallier *et al.* [18] said that the occurrence of high levels of Giardia cysts in raw water samples might require water utilities to apply treatment. Data indicate that disinfection as the only treatment for surface water sources is ineffective in preventing waterborne transmission of this organism [19]. For water treatment, G. lamblia cysts can inactivated in water with ozone at pH 7.0 [20].

The problem of contamination in bivalve shellfish in the seashore where the drained contaminated water is collected can also be seen similar to the case of Cryptosporidium spp [21]. Schets *et al.* [22] that the detection of Giardia in seashells destined for human consumption has implications for public health only when human pathogenic cysts that had preserved infectivity during their stay in a marine environment were present. Schets *et al.* [22] suggested that consumption of raw oysters from the Oosterschelde might occasionally lead to cases of gastro-intestinal illness. Gómez-Couso *et al.* [23] detected in mussels, river water and waste waters and stated the wide distribution of this enteropathogen in the environment and the potential risk to public health associated with the consumption of raw or undercooking bivalves and use of these estuaries for recreational purposes.

Free living ameba contamination in water

Free living ameba is an important human pathogen. Acanthameba keratitis caused by Acanthameba spp. and Naegleria meningoencephalitis caused by Naegleria spp. are the two most lethal free living ameba infections [24]. Contamination of free living ameba in the water reservoir is a great public health concern [24]. Free living ameba can be isolated from a variety of habitats including fresh water, thermal discharges of power plants, soil and sewage [25]. Contamination by free living ameba in natural hot springs may pose a significant health risk to people who use such water for recreation activities [26]. The contamination of free living ameba in water reservoir can be seen. However, the health threat is not as much as the two previously described parasite. There are some reports on contamination of free living ameba in hotspring water [27-28] and to manage the water contamination by free living ameba is a focus in management of hot spring pools for tourist purpose. The main concern on free living ameba contamination is the disease namely primary amebic meningoencephalitis [29]. There are some noted cases of this disease according to direct contact, not ingestion, to the contaminated water.

Guinea worm contamination in water

Guinea worm (*Dracunculus medinensis*), is a round worm parasitic worm that can be found in India and Africa [30-31]. It can enter the body via drinking water and migrates to break out through the skin [30-31]. Several local people in the risk area become infected when they drink water containing copepods (water fleas) that harbor infective stage larvae [30-31]. Stagnant sources of drinking water, such as ponds, cisterns, pools in dried up riverbeds, temporary hand-dug wells and step-wells, usually harbor populations of copepods and are the usual sites where infection is transmitted [30-31]. In disease endemic villages the prevalence ranges from 15% to 70% [32-34]. In 1986, there were upto 3.5 million cases in 20 different countries in Asia and Africa. In 2002 fewer than 55 000 cases were noted, from 13 African countries [32-34]. The biggest burden of Guinea worm disease at present occurs in Sudan, Ghana and Nigeria [32-34]. It should be noted that these 3 countries together sum for 93% of all cases worldwide, with Sudan reporting 73% of the cases [32-34].

Conclusion

This is a short review of some parasitic water borne diseases. It should conclude about the lack of water safety and the need of sanitation in developing countries. This conclusion could open on other waterborne diseases (other than parasitic ones), and the role of the medical teams in making people and authorities aware of the need of clean water for health.

2. SOIL CONTAMINATION WITH PATHOGENIC PARASITE IN THAILAND: A SUMMARY

Introduction

Soil contamination with pathogenic parasite is a big public health problem in tropical developing countries. Diseases transmitted by soil are common in many tropical areas, including Thailand. Several efforts for control of those diseases are in place [35]. Surveys of parasites in soil samples are practiced and a high prevalence of soil contamination is noted. There are many important soil-transmitted helminths in Thailand, i.e. hookworm, Ascaris, Trichuris and Strongyloides. In this article, the author summarized the prevalence of soil contamination with pathogenic parasite in Thailand.

Materials and methods

A.   Primary data

This study was designed as a descriptive retrospective study. A literature review on the papers concerning blood lead level among several risk occupations in Thailand was performed. The author performed the literature review from database of the published works cited in the Index Medicus and Science Citation Index using key word "soil" and "parasite". The reports that lacked English text or contained no complete data were excluded for further analysis.

B.   Statistical analysis

Descriptive statistics were used in analysis. For each report, the prevalence of soil contamination was extracted. The summarization to find overall prevalence was performed. In addition, the correlation between the prevalence and setting was also assessed using Chi-square test. All the statistical analyses in this study were made using SPSS 7.0 for Windows Program.

Results

According to the search there are 7 reports [36-43] covering 562 soil samples on soil parasitic contamination in Thailand (December 2007). The details of each study were presented in Table

1. Overall prevalence of contamination is equal to 9.3 %. There is no significant correlation between setting and prevalence.

Table 1. Reports of soil contamination with pathogenic parasite in Thailand.

Report	Setting	Number of soil samples	Prevalence
Maipanich *et al.* [36]	Southern	71	6.9 %
Maipanich *et al.* [37]	Southern	69	1.7 %
Waenlor *et al.* [38]	Northern	24	16.7 %
Wiwanitkit *et al.* [39]	Northern	100	17.0 %
Wiwanitkit *et al.* [40]	Central	30	6.0 %
Wiwanitkit *et al.* [41]	Central	175	5.7 %
Maipanich *et al.* [42]	Northern	29	25 %
Uga *et al.* [43]	Southern	64	21 %

*There are five main regions of Thailand: northern, northeastern, southern, eastern and central regions.

Discussion

Soil-transmitted helminthiosis has been posing a public health problem in Thailand for several decades. The diagnosis of parasitic infections depends on a high level of suspicion after a thorough history and physical examination, mindful of relapsing course of long incubation periods [44]. A helminthiosis control program under the responsibility of the Communicable Disease Control Department, Ministry of Public Health was introduced in 1971. The program of treatment with effective anthelmintic drugs, health education and improvement of environmental sanitation [45-46]. Despite these efforts, the prevalence rate of infection in all population groups remains significant with high re-infection rates in endemic areas.

According to this work, the author analyzed the data on parasitic contamination in Thailand. Of interest, as high as 9.3 % of soil samples pose pathogenic parasitic contamination. This rate is comparable to other tropical countries. Because Thailand is a tropical country, the problem of soil-transmitted helminthiosis is very difficult to eradicate. How to success in control should be the promotion of preventive behavior especially for wearing shoes and good toileting.

3. REFERENCES

1. Smith HV, Rose JB. Waterborne cryptosporidiosis: current status. Parasitol Today 1998 Jan; 14(1): 14-22.

2. Fayer R, Speer CA, Dubey J.P. The general biology of Cryptosporidium. In: Fayer R, ed. Cryptosporidium and Cryptosporidiosis. Boca Raton,FL : CRC Press, 1997; 1-42.

3. Girdwood RWA, Smith HV. Cryptosporidium. In: Robinson R, Batt C, Patel P, eds. Encyclopaedia of Food Microbiology, Academic Press: London, 1999; 487-497.

4. Griffiths JK. Human cryptosporidiosis: epidemiology, transmission, treatment and diagnosis. Adv.Parasitol 1998; 40 : 37-85.

5. Nichols RAB, Smith HV. Parasites: Cryptosporidium, Giardia and Cyclospora as foodborne pathogens. In: C. de W. Blackburn and P.J. McClure, Editors, Foodborne Pathogens. Hazards, Risk Analysis and Control, Woodhead Publishing Ltd., Cambridge, UK (2001), pp. 453-478.

6. Robertson LJ, Gjerde B. Isolation and enumeration of Giardia cysts, cryptosporidium oocysts, and Ascaris eggs from fruits and vegetables. J Food Prot. 2000 Jun; 63(6): 775-8.

7. Rose JB, Slifko TR. Giardia, Cryptosporidium, and Cyclospora and their impact on foods: a review. J Food Prot. 1999 Sep; 62(9): 1059-70.

8. Fayer R, Dubey JP, Lindsay DS. Zoonotic protozoa: from land to sea. Trends Parasitol 2004 Nov; 20(11): 531-6.

9. Fayer R, Trout JM, Lewis EJ, Santin M, Zhou L, Lal AA, Xiao L. Contamination of Atlantic coast commercial shellfish with Cryptosporidium, Parasitol Res. 2003 Jan; 89(2): 141-5.

10.   Melo PC, Teodosio J, Reis J, Duarte A, Costa JC, Fonseca IP. Cryptosporidium spp. in freshwater bivalves in Portugal. J Eukaryot Microbiol 2006; 53 Suppl 1: S28-9.

11.   Miller WA, Atwill ER, Gardner IA, Miller MA, Fritz HM, Hedrick RP, Melli AC, Barnes NM, Conrad PA. Clams (Corbicula fluminea) as bioindicators of fecal contamination with Cryptosporidium and Giardia spp. in freshwater ecosystems in California. Int J Parasitol 2005 May; 35(6): 673-84.

12.   Gómez-Couso H, Méndez-Hermida F, Ares-Mazás E. Levels of detection of Cryptosporidium oocysts in mussels (Mytilus galloprovincialis) by IFA and PCR methods. Vet Parasitol 2006 Oct 10; 141(1-2): 60-5.

13.   Gómez-Couso H, Méndez-Hermida F, Castro-Hermida JA, Ares-Mazás E. Giardia in shellfish-farming areas: detection in mussels, river water and waste waters. Vet Parasitol 2005 Oct 10; 133(1): 13-8.

14.   Wolfe MS. Giardiasis. N Engl J Med 1978 Feb 9; 298(6): 319-21.

15.   Anceno AJ, Ozaki M, Yen Nga DD, Chuluun B, Shipin OV. Canal networks as extended waste stabilization ponds: fate of pathogens in constructed waterways in Pathumthani Province, Thailand. Canal networks as extended waste stabilization ponds: fate of pathogens in constructed waterways in Pathumthani Province, Thailand. Water Sci Technol. 2007; 55(11): 143-56.

16.   Uga S, Kunaruk N, Rai SK, Watanabe M. Cryptosporidium infection in HIV-seropositive and seronegative populations in southern Thailand. Southeast Asian J Trop Med Public Health 1998; 29 (1): 100-4.

17.   Kent GP, Greenspan JR, Herndon JL, Mofenson LM, Harris JA, Eng TR, Waskin HA. Epidemic giardiasis caused by a contaminated public water supply. Am J Public Health 1988 Feb; 78(2): 139-43.

18.   LeChevallier MW, Norton WD, Lee RG. Occurrence of Giardia and Cryptosporidium spp. in surface water supplies. Appl Environ Microbiol 1991 Sep; 57(9): 2610-6.

19.   Craun GF. Waterborne giardiasis in the United States: a review. Am J Public Health 1979 Aug; 69(8): 817-9.

20.   Wickramanayake GB, Rubin AJ, Sproul OJ. Inactivation of Giardia lamblia cysts with ozone. Appl Environ Microbiol 1984 Sep; 48(3): 671-2.

21.   Giangaspero A. Giardia. Cryptosporidium and the spectre of zoonosis: the Italian experience from land to sea. Parassitologia 2006 Jun; 48(1-2): 95-100.

22.   Schets FM, van den Berg HH, Engels GB, Lodder WJ, de Roda Husman AM. Cryptosporidium and Giardia in commercial and non-commercial oysters (Crassostrea gigas) and water from the Oosterschelde, The Netherlands.

23.   Gomez-Bautista M, Ortega-Mora LM, Tabares E, Lopez-Rodas V, Costas E. Detection of infectious Cryptosporidium parvum oocysts in mussels (Mytilus galloprovincialis) and cockles (Cerastoderma edule). Appl Environ Microbiol 2000 May; 66(5): 1866-70.

24.   Schuster FL, Visvesvara GS. Free-living amoebae as opportunistic and non-opportunistic pathogens of humans and animals. Int J Parasitol 2004 Aug; 34(9): 1001-27.

25.   Visvesvara GS, Stehr-Green JK. Epidemiology of free-living ameba infections. J Protozool 1990 Jul-Aug; 37(4): 25S-33S.

26.   Lekkla A, Sutthikornchai C, Bovornkitti S, Sukthana Y. Free-living ameba contamination in natural hot springs in Thailand. Southeast Asian J Trop Med Public Health 2005; 36 Suppl 4: 5-9.

27.   Cursons R, Sleigh J, Hood D, Pullon D. A case of primary amoebic meningoencephalitis: North Island, New Zealand. N Z Med J 2003 Dec 12; 116(1187): U712.

28.   Ellis-Pegler R. Primary amoebic meningoencephalitis--rare and lethal. N Z Med J 2003 Dec 12; 116(1187): U705.

29.   Wiwanitkit V. Review of clinical presentations in Thai patients with primary amoebic meningoencephalitis. MedGenMed 2004 Mar 8; 6(1): 2.

30.   Greenaway C. Dracunculiasis (Guinea worm disease) CMAJ 2004; 170: 495-500.

      Int J Food Microbiol 2007 Jan 25; 113(2): 189-94.

31.   Kyei-faried S, Appiah-denkyira E, Brenya D, Akuamoa-Boateng A, Visser I. The role of community-based surveillance in health outcomes measurement. Ghana Med J 2006; 40: 26-30.

32.   Aylward RB, Birmingham M. The human story. BMJ 2005; 331; 1261-1262.

33.   MacDonald R. Access to clean water in rural Africa is inadequate. BMJ 2005; 331: 70.

34.   Tumwine JK. Clean drinking water for homes in Africa and other less developed countries. BMJ 2005; 331; 468-469.

35.   Huttly SR. The impact of inadequate sanitary conditions on health in developing countries. World Health Stat Q 1990; 43: 118-26.

36.   Maipanich W, Waikagul J, Pahuchon W, Muennoo C, Visiessuk K. Contamination of soil-transmitted helminth eggs in soil samples from Nakhon Si Thammarat Province. J Trop Med Parasitol 1995; 18: 22-30.

37.   Maipanich W, Pahuchon W, Visiessuk K, Nontasut P, Waikagul J. Soil-transmitted helminths in human host and soil pollution after quaternary treatment. J Trop Med Parasitol 1996; 1: 48-54.

38.   Waenlor W, Wiwanitkit V, Suyaphan A. Study of soil contamination with geohelminths in a rural Karen village, Nahongtai. Chula Med J 2002; 46: 941-947.

39.   Wiwanitkit V, Waenlor W, Suyaphan A. Contamination of soil with parasites in a tropical hilltribe village in Northern Thailand. Trop Doct 2003; 33: 180-2.

40.   Wiwanitkit V, Waenlor W. Contamination of soil with parasites in a Thai hospital. Am J Infect Control 2005; 33: 374-5.

41.   Maipanich W, Itiponpanya N, Sukosol T, Rojekittikhun W, Pubampen S, Sa-nguankiat S, Siripanth C, Juntanavivat C, Incheang S. J Trop Med Parasitol 2002 ; 25,1 : 30-37.

42.   Wiwanitkit V, Waenlor W. The frequency rate of Toxocara species contamination in soil samples from public yards in a urban area "Payathai," Bangkok, Thailand. Rev Inst Med Trop Sao Paulo 2004; 46: 113-114.

43.   Uga S, Nagnaen W, Chongsuvivatwong V. Contamination of soil with parasite eggs and oocysts in southern Thailand. Southeast Asian J Trop Med Public Health 1997; 28 Suppl 3: 14-7.

44.   Cutrona AF, Rothschild BM. Recognition and treatment of endemic and travel-acquire parasitosis. Compr Ther 1994; 20: 445-58.

45.   Shrestha A, Rai SK, Basnyat SR, Rai CK, Shakya B. Soil transmitted helminthiasis in Kathmandu, Nepal. Nepal Med Coll J 2007 Sep; 9(3): 166-9.

46.   Rai SK, Uga S, Ono K, Rai G, Matsumura T. Contamination of soil with helminth parasite eggs in Nepal. Southeast Asian J Trop Med Public Health 2000 Jun; 31(2): 388-93.

CHAPTER 4

SUCCESSFUL OF CONTROL PROGRAM FOR ENTEROBIASIS AMONG HILLTRIBERS IN A RURAL COMMUNITY, NORTHERN THAILAND

Viroj Wiwanitkit[1] and Akkaradej Suyaphan[2]

[1]*Wiwanitkit House, Bangkhae, Bangkok Thailand 10160;*

[2]*Hospital Administrator, Mae Jam Hospital, Chiangmai Thailand*

Address correspondence to: Professor Viroj Wiwanitkit, Wiwanitkit House, Bangkhae, Bangkok Thailand 10160 Email: wviroj@yahoo.com

Abstract: *Enterobius vermicularis* is an important helminthic infection among children in rural areas of developing countries. In our previous reports, a high prevalence of enterobiasis among the children in the far rural community, Mae Suk, Northern Thailand was noted. An active control program for enterobiasis in our community is set and distribution of antihelminthic drugs and a longitudinal follow-up to assess the effectiveness of our control program was performed. Here, the author reports a dramatic decrease of the prevalence of enterobiasis in this rural area.

Keywords: enterobiasis, triber, control.

1. INTRODUCTION

Enterobius vermicularis is an important helminthic infection among children in rural areas of developing countries. The most typical symptom is perianal pruritus, especially at night, which may lead to excoriations [1-2]. This infection affects the general health as well as the intelligence of the infected children.[3-4]. The prevalence of enterobiasis among Thai children has dramatically decreased in big cities, however, high prevalence among the children in far rural areas can be expected.

In our previous reports, a high prevalence of enterobiasis among the children in the far rural community, Mae Suk, Northern Thailand was noted. The noted prevalence among the hilltribers in the rural community is upto 40 % [5]. Hence, enterobiasis is a very important infectious disease in this rural setting. An active control program for enterobiasis in our community is set and distribution of antihelminthic drugs and a longitudinal follow-up to assess the effectiveness of our control program was performed. Here, the author reports a dramatically decrease of the prevalence of enterobiasis in this rural area.

2. MATERIALS AND METHODS

Background

In 2001, the team visited the hilltribe villages of the Mae Suk District, Chiangmai Province. The setting is the rural district of Thailand, surrounded by hills, and a number of hilltribers have settled here. Its location is about 800 km from Bangkok, the capital of Thailand. All 291 children (123 males, 168 females) from 10 villages in this district were tested for the presence of E vermicularis egg was performed by perianal tape examination [5]. Of the total 291 children examined an overall infection rate of E vermicularis of 41.6% was derived [5].

Control program

The local hospital along with the local public health center performed a continuous health education as well as antihelminthic drug distribution to the villagers. The Thai-tribal language translator was used in all of the communication. The local people in this area were willing to participate in the control program. The evaluation of the control program was set at 6 months after the starting.

Measurement of the prevalence of enterobiasis after control program

In February 2002, the team visit the villages again and the repeat procedure for examination of eneterobiasis among the children. All specimen collections were performed at the subjects' homes between 6: 00 and 8: 00 AM. All collected samples were sent for identification of the parasite under light microscope at the nearest laboratory, Mae Jam Hospital, Chiangmai, by the medical technologist teams.

3. RESULTS

According to our study to evaluate the successful of the program, we got 178 subjects (70 males and 108 females) for perianal tape examination. The lost 113 subjects are due to the migrating to other setting as the nature of hill tribers. Of overall 178 subjects, the presence of E vermicularis infection was detected in 56 cases, giving infection rate equal to 31.5 %. To make a comparison to the pre-control prevalence, our team tried to match the cases without dropping out and the post-control prevalence is presented in Table 1.

Table 1. The rate of *E vermicularis* infection after the control program.

Subjects	Pre-control		Post-control	
	Number of infected cases	%	Number of infected cases	%
Males (n = 70)	28	40.0	20	28.6
Females (n = 108)	44	40.7	36	33.3

4. DISCUSSION

One of the possible explanations for very high prevalence of enterobiasis among hilltribers is that these tribers can be considered as minorities, lacking in primary healthcare [5]. Their daily lifestyle is the same as their ancestors, lacking of facilities. Here, the authors report the result of a control program for enterobiasis among the hilltribers. According to this report, a favorable result, decreasing of the infection rate can be derived.

The overall infection rate, without considering of dropping out, decrease from 41.6 % to 31.5 %. Even though matching for the case after dropping out, the similar trend of decrease (40.4% to 31.5%; Table 1) can be seen. Of interest, although there are many reports on the prevalence survey of enterobiasis among rural communities in tropical countries including Thailand there are only a few reports on the success of the control program. In addition, the control program among the tribers is very hard. Here, a high rate of dropping out due to migrant nature of the tribers is a big problem. The dropped out cases might be a reservoir of disease to new community, brining a new problem to the new setting. This can also imply the importance of travel medicine.

Although the rate after control program is still high our team hope that if the control program is continuously introduce to the community and the control of migration is successful, more lowering of the rate can be derived. Also, it should be considered for the nature of the disease that the re-infection can easily occurs [1-2] and this can affect the effectiveness of mass medication. These reasons can confirm the necessary of the continuous control. However, this study can support the report of Lohiya *et al.* that mass medication of residents with enterobiasis and their contacts was beneficial, harmless, and cost effective [6].

5. ACKNOWLEDGEMENT

The authors thank all public health officers in all surveyed villages. We are thankful to Mr. Sahlae Por, the Thai-tribal language translator for our team. Also, the authors would like to give thank to Surasith Thiamtip, Head of District Public Health Officer, Mae Jam District who support all of the program. Finally, the author would like to acknowledge Tisak Chaisalee,

Jamsai Suwansaksri and Attapon Tukaew who are our collaborators in the early community creening.

6. REFERENCES

1. Finn L. Threadworm infections. Community Nurse 1996; 2: 39.

2. Grencis RK, Cooper ES. Enterobius, trichuris, capillaria, and hookworm including ancylostoma caninum. Gastroenterol Clin North Am 1996; 25: 579-597.

3. Avolio L, Avoltini V, Ceffa F, Bragheri R. Perianal granuloma caused by Enterobius vermicularis: report of a new observation and review of the literature. J Pediatr. 1998; 132: 1055-1056.

4. Bahader SM, Ali GS, Shaalan AH, Khalil HM, Khalil NM. Effects of Enterobius vermicularis infection on intelligence quotient (IQ) and anthropometric measurements of Egyptian rural children. J Egypt Soc Parasitol 1995; 25: 183-194.

5. Chaisalee T, Tukaew A, Wiwanitkit V, Suyaphun A, Thiamtip S, Suwansaksri J. Very high prevalence of enterobiasis among the hilltribal children in rural district "Mae Suk," Thailand. MedGenMed 2004; 6: 5.

6. Lohiya GS, Tan-Figueroa L, Crinella FM, Lohiya S. Epidemiology and control of enterobiasis in a developmental center. West J Med 2000; 172: 305-8.

CHAPTER 5

OVERVIEW OF CONJUNCTIVITIS IN THAILAND

Kunakorn Atchaneeyasakul[1] and Viroj Wiwanitkit[2]

[1]Faculty of Medicine, Chulalongkorn University, Bangkok Thailand 10330;

[2]Wiwanitkit House, Bangkhae, Bangkok Thailand 10160

Address correspondence to: Professor Viroj Wiwanitkit, Wiwanitkit House, Bangkhae, Bangkok Thailand 10160 Email: wviroj@yahoo.com

Abstract: Conjunctivitis is an infectious disease of the eye which is very common in Thailand. The disease can spread widely and especially during the rainy season in Thailand. The authors performed a literature review on the reports of Conjunctivitis outbreak in Thailand in order to summarize the outbreak information. A literature review of the papers concerning Conjunctivitis outbreak in Thailand was performed using the database of published works cited in the Index Medicus and Science Citation index. The literature review focused mainly on all conjunctivitis outbreaks that have been published. The reported location of the outbreak in the literature usually occurred in central Thailand mostly in the capital city, Bangkok. Some outbreaks can be found in other parts of Thailand such as the Northeastern Thailand. The time of outbreak is usually around August which is around the rainy season in Thailand. There is no significant difference of the infection between male and female. The calculated overall mean age of patients is 16 years which is the school age. Conjunctivitis is a common eye infection caused by many kinds of organisms which is highly contagious and is able to spread just by contact. The disease is not severe and can be treated by topical antibiotics. However it is much wise to keep the infection from spreading by keeping the patients away from social for about a week.

Keywords: conjunctivitis, Thailand.

1. INTRODUCTION

Conjunctivitis is an inflammation of the conjunctiva, most commonly owing to an allergic reaction or an infection (usually bacterial, such as fecal matter contaminating the eye, or viral). Redness, irritation and watering of the eyes are common symptoms to all forms of conjunctivitis. The first reported outbreak of conjunctivitis occurred in Ghana and Nigeria, Africa in the year 1969 and later on spread throughout Africa. In the year 1970, the disease spread on to Indonesia and Singapore, finally spreading onward to Panama. Finally, from August to October of 1981, the disease finally spread worldwide.

The first report on an outbreak was published in 1971. This disease is mainly caused by virus and can be spread easily by personal contact. The incubation period is only 24-48 hrs. The disease usually lasts not longer than 2 weeks. Rainy season is common for conjunctivitis in Thailand starting from June to middle period of November [1-11]. In this work, the authors summarized the epidemic of conjunctivitis outbreak in Thailand.

2. MATERIALS AND METHODS

This study was designed as a descriptive retrospective study. A literature review of the papers concerning conjunctivitis outbreak in Thailand was performed, using the database of published works cited in the Index Medicus and Science Citation index. Local reports available in the local database, Thai Index Medicus, are also searched. The literature review focused mainly on all conjunctivitis outbreaks that have been published.

There are currently 11 published works on conjunctivitis available in the Index Medicus and Science Citation index. The published works contain information on each conjunctivitis outbreak that occurred in a particular area of study. The information includes the location of the outbreak, number of patients known, time of the outbreak, mean age of patients, and diagnosis method, which all differ in each literature. Then the authors gathered all the information to process it in to one simple table for comparing the results from each outbreak.

3. RESULTS

According to this study, there have been a total of 11 outbreaks published in 11 literatures gathered (Table 1). However, some of the published information excluded sex, age, and number of actual patients (3 of 11 did not have age listed, 5 of 11 did not identify the sex of patients, and 1 of 11 excluded the number of patients). The remaining results that have been gathered can be summarized into the following paragraphs.

The reported location of the outbreak in the literature was usually in central Thailand mostly in the capital city, Bangkok. Some outbreaks can be found in other parts of Thailand such as the Northeastern Thailand. The information interpreted from the literature is that conjunctivitis can often spread in highly populated area. The time of outbreak is usually around August which falls in the rainy season in Thailand. There is no significant difference of the infection between males and females. The number of infected person in all the outbreaks in all the journals sums up to 5381 people in entire Thailand. From the 4815 cases with sex listed it sums up to 2536 males and 2216 females.

The calculated overall mean age of patients is 16 years which is the school age (minimum = 8 years old, maximum = 58 years old, SD = 17.2 years). One of the papers quote that "The infection often spread in populated places such as school or factory and happens when the same restrooms are used by all."[7] The methods of diagnosis mainly used in the papers are serologic investigation and eye swab culture. Percentages of positive cultures, serology and viral isolation are 16.7 % (2/12), 32.1 % (42/131) and 100 % (9/9), respectively. Only some papers have symptoms description which includes eye irritation, pain, subconjunctival hemorrhage, rash, and preauricular lymphadenopathy.1 Most of the infection in Thailand often occurred form Coxsakievirus A type 24 [8-10] and Enterovirus type 70 [8].

4. DISCUSSION

Conjuctivitis is a common eye infection caused by many kinds of organisms which is highly contagious and is able to spread just by contact. The disease is not severe and can be treated by topical antibiotics. However, it is much wise to keep the infection from spreading by keeping the patients away from social for about a week. Here, the authors have overviewed viral conjunctivitis outbreak in Thailand.

An outbreak of acute hemorrhagic conjunctivitis that occurred in Maharashtra and Gujarat, states of India during August-September 2003 was caused by Coxsakievirus A type 24 for which the time of outbreak and infectious organism is also similar to Thailand's conjunctivitis outbreak. The method of diagnosis used in the paper [12] was also similar to a Thai paper which discussed viral isolation from eye swab.

An outbreak of acute hemorrhagic conjunctivitis occurred in French Guiana between April and July 2003, with approximately 6,000 cases in the two major cities Kourou and Cayenne [13]. The infectious organism which is the cause of this outbreak is also Coxakievirus A type 2413. The time of outbreak is at around the time of summer [13]. Viral isolation from eye swab is also used. The main reason for the spread of conjunctivitis is that the same type of virus from Thailand that caused the disease was introduced from Asia [12-14] and it rapidly spread into the Caribbean [15-16], where the infection disappeared after a few months.

Two outbreaks of acute hemorrhagic conjunctivitis that occurred in the Democratic Republic of the Congo and in Morocco [17] in the summers of 2003 and 2004 were reported. Virus was isolated from the conjunctival swabs of 30 Congolese and 20 Moroccan patients. The viruses could be identified as coxsackie A24 variants. From DNA investigation, it can be found that the virus is very similar to Asian virus, thus proving their worldwide spread [18-19].

There is no specific treatment for conjunctivitis except for symptomatic treatment and prevention of infection. Common medication is antibiotic and steroidal drugs. Conclusively, the outbreaks of viral conjunctivitis in Thailand are usually due to Coxsakievirus A type 24 and Enterovirus type 70. The time of outbreak is usually in rainy season.

Table 1. Overview of conjunctivitis outbreak in Thailand.

No.	Authors	Location of outbreak	Time of outbreak	Number of patients (M,F)	Mean age	Method in diagnosis
1	Kosupat S. Thampaolo S. 1990	Nakhonpathom, Central Thailand	August	128 (80,48)	21	Culture Serology
2	Rerkgarm S. Narkkroun J. 1985	Ubonrajathanee, Northeastern Thailand	August	82 (82,0)	18	Serology
3	Prablipudlung A. Saichur S. Gulyaganon T. Sukulrachata M. Harnpanich W. Wilaiprasert S. 1980	Khonkhan, Northeastern Thailand	August	138 (86,52)	20	Culture Microscopy
4	Thongcharoen P. Wasi C. Pimolpan V. Panpatana P. 1971-1975	Bangkok, Central Thailand	July	133	NA	Culture Serology Viral isolation
5	Thongcharoen P. Jatikavanij V. Wasi C. Pimolpan V. Panpatana P. 1971	Bangkok, Central Thailand	August	4157 (1978, 2116)	14	Culture Serology Viral isolation
6	Dumavibhat P. Thongcharoen P. Jatikavanij V. Wasi C. Pimolpan V. Panpatana P. 1971	Bangkok, Central Thailand	June	2105 (988, 1117)	19	Culture Serology Viral isolation
7	Petwanich A. 1986-1988	Bangkok, Central Thailand	July	107	NA	NA
8	Jayavasu C. Santiswadinont P. Sagnuanwong S. 1975	Central Thailand	NA	NA	NA	Culture Serology Viral isolation
9	Aekwittayopas A. 1992	Nakhonratchasima, Northeastern Thailand	September	310 (310,0)	17	Serology
10	Thai CDC. 1994	Nakhonpathom, Central Thailand	August	409	13	Serology
11	Sukgawee R. 1996	Bangkok, Central Thailand	March	50	34	Viral isolation Serology

NA = not applicable

5. REFERENES

1.   Kosupat S, Thampaolo S. Surveillace of conjunctivitis outbreak in Kasetsart University, Kampangsan campus, Nakhon Prathom province. J Soc Acad PDRH 1990; 7: 34-45.

2.   Rerkgarm S, Narkkroun J. Repor of the investigation of the acute hemorrhagic conjunctivitis outbreak at Wat Thung Sri Muang, Ubonrajathanee. Med J Ubon Hosp 1985; 6: 79-84.

3.   Prablipudlung A, Saichur S, Gulyaganon T, Sukulrachata M, Harnpanich W, Wilaiprasert S. Etiology of conjunctivitis in Khonkhan university hospital. Khonkaen Univ Health Sci Cent Bull 1980; 6: 123-133.

4.   Thongcharoen P, Wasi C, Pimolpan V, Panpatana P. Etiologic studies on acute hemorrhagic conjunctivitis in Thailand 1971-1975. J Med Assoc Thai 1978; 61: 195-201.

5.   Thongcharoen P, Jatikavanij V, Wasi C, Pimolpan V, Panpatana P. An outbreak of acute hemorrhagic conjunctivitis in Thailand epidemiologic investigation. J Med Assoc Thai 1974; 57: 248-251.

6.   Dumavibhat P, Thongcharoen P, Jatikavanij V, Wasi C, Pimolpan V, Panpatana P. An outbreak of acute hemorrhagic conjunctivitis in Thailand clinical observation. J Med Assoc Thai 1977; 56: 267-272.

7.   Petwanich A. Acute hemorrhagic conjunctivitis. Clinic 1988; 4: 611-613.

8.   Jayavasu C, Santiswadinont P, Sagnuanwong S. An enteroviruses associated with an epidemic of the acute haemorrhagic conjunctivitis in Thailand 1975. Bull Dept Med Sci 1977; 19: 207-215.

9.   Aekwittayopas A. Report of investigation of conjunctivitis outbreak in juvenile protection facility in Nakhonratchasima 8-9 October 1992. W Epidemiol Surveil Rep 1994; 25: 117-120, 126-129.

10.   Thai CDC. Report of investigation of conjunctivitis outbreak in a secondary school in Sampran Nakhon prathom. W Epidemiol Surveil Rep 1995; 26: 330-334, 341-342.

11.   Sukgawee R. Investigation of conjunctivitis in a village in Bungkum Bangkok 6-15 March 1996. Month Epidemiol Surveil Rep 1996; 5: 1-4, 37-39.

12.   Gopalkrishna V, Patil PR, Kolhapure RM, Bilaiya H, Fulmali PV, Deolankar RP. Outbreak of acute hemorrhagic conjunctivitis in Maharashtra and Gujarat states of India, caused by Coxsackie virus A-24 variant. J Med Virol. 2007; 79: 748-53.

13.   Dussart P, Cartet G, Huguet P, Lévêque N, Hajjar C, Morvan J, Vanderkerckhove J, Ferret K, Lina B, Chomel JJ, Norder H. Outbreak of acute hemorrhagic conjunctivitis in French Guiana and West Indies caused by coxsackievirus A24 variant: phylogenetic analysis reveals Asian import. J Med Virol. 2005; 75: 559-65.

14.   Yin-Murphy M, Baharuddin-Ishak, Phoon MC, Chow VT. A recent epidemic of Coxsackie virus type A24 acute haemorrhagic conjunctivitis in Singapore. Br J Ophthalmol 1986; 70: 869-73.

15.   Rédon IA, Lago PJ, Pérez LR, Puentes P, Corredor MB. Outbreak of acute haemorrhagic conjunctivitis in Cuba. Mem Inst Oswaldo Cruz 1999; 94: 467-8.

16.   Centers for Disease Control and Prevention (CDC). Acute hemorrhagic conjunctivitis outbreak caused by Coxsackievirus A24--Puerto Rico, 2003. MMWR Morb Mortal Wkly Rep 2004; 53: 632-4.

17.   Nejmi S, Gaudin OG, Chomel JJ, Baaj A, Sohier R, Bosshard S. Isolation of a virus responsible for an outbreak of acute haemorrhagic conjunctivitis in Morocco. J Hyg (Lond) 1974; 72: 181-3.

18.   Ishiko H, Takeda N, Miyamura K, Kato N, Tanimura M, Lin KH, Yin-Murphy M, Tam JS, Mu GF, Yamazaki S. Phylogenetic analysis of a coxsackievirus A24 variant: the most recent worldwide pandemic was caused by progenies of a virus prevalent around 1981. Virology 1992; 187: 748-59.

19.   Kew OM, Nottay BK, Hatch MH, Hierholzer JC, Obijeski JF. Oligonucleotide fingerprint analysis of enterovirus 70 isolates from the 1980 to 1981 pandemic of acute hemorrhagic conjunctivitis: evidence for a close genetic relationship among Asian and American strains. Infect Immun 1983; 41: 631-5.

CHAPTER 6

HEMAGGLUTININ GENE OF BIRD FLU VIRUS IN THAILAND: A VARIATION OF THEIR ENCODING PROTEINS

Viroj Wiwanitkit[1]

[1]Wiwanitkit House, Bangkhae, Bangkok Thailand 10160

Address correspondence to: Professor Viroj Wiwanitkit, Wiwanitkit House, Bangkhae, Bangkok Thailand 10160 Email: wviroj@yahoo.com

Abstract: Background: Bird flu or avian flu, caused by H5N1 virus, is a new emerging infectious disease. It is noted that this H5N1 virus jumped the species barrier and caused severe disease with high mortality in humans in Vietnam and Thailand. Many were reported noted on nucleotide for HA of H5N1 in Thailand. However, there is no comparison on the structure of the protein encoded by the isolated HA in Thailand.

Method: Here, the author performed this study to compare the secondary and tertiary structures of the isolated HA from different sources in Thailand. The author used a bioinformatic technique to predict the secondary and tertiary structures of HA of H5N1 isolated in Thailand.

Result: Using NNPREDICT and CPHmodels 2.0 servers, the calculation for secondary and tertiary structures of H5N1 of HA isolated in Thailand was performed. The predicted structures of all 20 HA are same.

Conclusion: The structures of H5N1 derived from natural and non-natural hosts of virus are same. This implies that the mutation might not be the important factor leading to the cross species infection in Thailand but the individual defect of non-avian host might be the possible factor.

Keywords: bird flu, Thailand, HA, structure, mutation.

1. INTRODUCTION

Bird flu or avian flu, caused by H5N1 virus, is a new emerging infectious disease. There has been worldwide situation regarding avian influenza infections in poultry from 1997. It is noted that this H5N1 virus jumped the species barrier and caused severe disease with high mortality in humans in Vietnam, Thailand and other countries. Most infected cases usually developed progressive pneumonia with acute respiratory distress syndrome and consequently died. Mutation of the virus is believed to be an important factor that can bring the pandemic of bird flu. Trampuz *et al.* said that the widespread epidemic of bird flu in avians increases the likelihood for mutational events and genetic reassortment [1]. Monitoring of mutational events becomes an important measure for infection control of bird flu [1-2].

There are many noted codons of nucleotide for HA of H5N1 in Thailand. Puthavathana *et al.* found that nucleotides of the viruses in Thailand were similar to those of the chicken virus and other H5N1 viruses from Hong Kong [3]. However, there is no comparison on the structure of the protein encoded by the isolated HA in Thailand. Here, the author performed this study to compare the secondary and tertiary structures of the isolated HA from different sources in Thailand.

2. METHODS

A.   Data mining for the nucleotides of HA of H5N1 in Thailand

The database Pubmed was used for data mining of the nucleotide and amino acid sequences for HA of H5N1 isolated in Thailand. Only complete sequences were included for further study.

B.   Structure modeling

The author performs protein secondary structure predictions of HA from its primary sequence using NNPREDICT server [4]. Also, The author performs protein tertiary structure predictions of HA from its primary sequence using CPHmodels 2.0 server [5]. The calculated secondary and tertiary structures were presented and compared.

3. RESULTS

A.   Sequence of HA in H5N1

From searching of the database PubMed, 20 complete sequences of H5N1 of HA isolated in Thailand was derived as shown in Table 1 (in February 2006).

Table 1. Complete sequences of H5N1 of HA isolated in Thailand.

Code	Description	Natural host
DQ334776	(A/chicken/Thailand/Nontaburi/CK-162/2005(H5N1))	Yes
DQ334778	(A/quail/Thailand/Nakhon Pathom/QA-161/2005(H5N1))	Yes
DQ334760	(A/chicken/Thailand/Kanchanaburi/CK-160/2005(H5N1))	Yes
AY972541	(A/tiger/Thailand/CU-T6/04(H5N1))	No
AY972539	(A/tiger/Thailand/CU-T4/04(H5N1))	No
AY646175	(A/leopard/Suphanburi/Thailand/Leo-1/04(H5N1))	No
AY972567	(A/tiger/Suphanburi/Thailand/Ti-1/04(H5N1))	No
AY555153	(A/Thailand/2(SP-33)/2004(H5N1))	No
DQ236085	(A/pigeon/Thailand/KU-03/04(H5N1))	Yes
DQ236077	(A/cat/Thailand/KU-02/04(H5N1))	No
DQ083585	(A/Mynas/Ranong/Thailand/CU-209/04(H5N1))	Yes
DQ083584	(A/sparrow/Phang-Nga/Thailand/CU-203/04(H5N1))	Yes
DQ083583	(A/pigeon/Samut Prakan/Thailand/CU-202/04(H5N1))	Yes
DQ083578	(A/chicken/Ratchaburi/Thailand/CU-68/04(H5N1))	Yes
DQ083573	(A/white peafowl/Bangkok/Thailand/CU-29/04(H5N1))	Yes
DQ083565	(A/chicken/Saraburi/Thailand/CU-17/04(H5N1))	Yes
DQ083564	(A/white peafowl/Bangkok/Thailand/CU-16/04(H5N1))	Yes
DQ083563	(A/crow/Bangkok/Thailand/CU-15/04(H5N1))	Yes
DQ083551	(A/chicken/Bangkok/Thailand/CU-3/04(H5N1))	Yes
DQ076201	(A/Ck/Thailand/73/2004(H5N1))	Yes

B.   Structure modeling

Using NNPREDICT server, the calculation for secondary structure of H5N1 of HA isolated in Thailand was performed. Using CPHmodels 2.0 server, the calculation for tertiary structure of H5N1 of HA isolated in Thailand was performed. The predicted structures of all 20 HA are same. The predicted secondary and tertiary structures are shown in Figure 1 and 2, respectively.

```
--HHHEHHHHHHE-----EEEEE--------H-HHHHH---E--H-HHHHH---------
-----EE----HH------------------EHHH--------------HHHHHHH
HHHH------EEE-----------E-------------HHHHHHHH------EEEE---
------HHHEEE-------HHHH------EEEEE----------HHH---------
-EEEEEEH-------E---------HHHHHHE------HE-----------------
-------E----------------HHHHE--------HHHH-----EEHHE-EEH---
--EE---E------------------H-HH---H-----EHH----HHHHHHHHHHHHH
HHHHHH---HHH-HHEHHHHHHHHHHHHHH-------------HHHHHHHH---HH--
--HHHEE------HHHH-----------HH-HHHHHHH----E-E--HEEEEEEEEEHH
HHHHHHEHHH---EEEE-------EE—
```

Figure 1. Predicted secondary structures of H5N1 of HA isolated in Thailand

(Secondary structure prediction: H = helix, E = strand,-= no prediction).

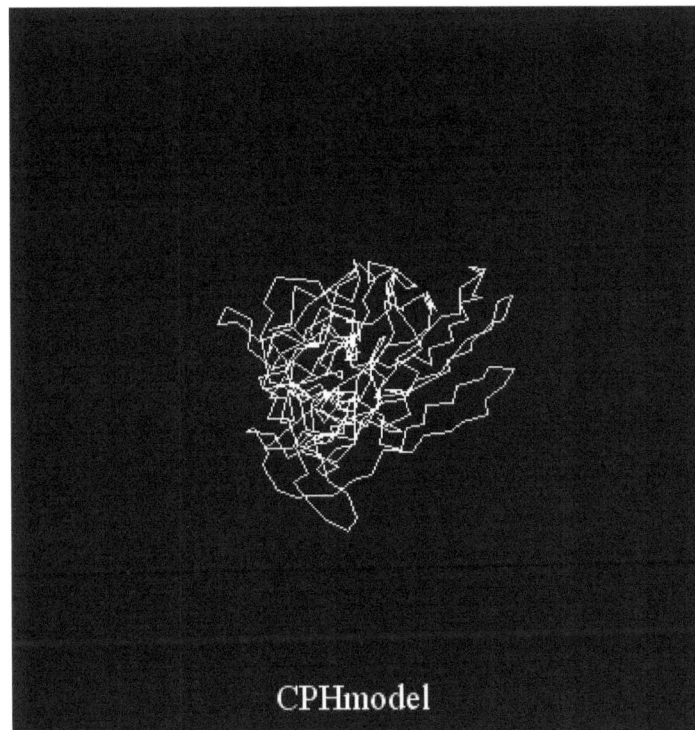

Figure 2. Predicted tertiary structures of H5N1 of HA isolated in Thailand.

4. DISCUSSION

Bird flu is an emerging infectious disease. Presently, the possibility of panendemic of bird flu around the world is a main discussed topic in public health.

Mutation within the genome of H5N1 is believed to be a possible factor contributing to emerging of this disease [6-7]. From genome analysis, Puthavathana *et al.* found that the Thailand viruses contained more avian-specific residues than the 1997 Hong Kong H5N1 viruses [3]. They suggested that the virus might have adapted to allow a more efficient spread in avian species [3].

However, based on the principle of molecular biology, only the mutation of nucleotide does not mean the alternation of expression, which implies the infectivity in this case. The mutation may be a silent one or can cause structural aberration of specific encoded protein, which can lead to alteration of protein expression. Here, the author used a bioinformatic technique to predict the secondary and tertiary structures of the HA of H5N1 isolated in Thailand. Of interest, the structures of H5N1 derived from natural and non-natural hosts of virus are same. This implies that the mutation might not be the important factor leading to· the cross species infection in Thailand but the individual defect of non-avian host might be the possible factor.

5. REFERENCES

1.   Trampuz A, Prabhu RM, Smith TF, Baddour LM. Avian influenza: a new pandemic threat? Mayo Clin Proc 2004; 79: 523-30

2.   Viseshakul N, Thanawongnuwech R, Amonsin A, Suradhat S, Payungporn S, Keawchareon J, Oraveerakul K, Wongyanin P, Plitkul S, Theamboonlers A, Poovorawan Y. The genome sequence analysis of H5N1 avian influenza A virus isolated from the outbreak among poultry populations in Thailand. Virology 2004; 328: 169-76.

3.   Puthavathana P, Auewarakul P, Charoenying PC, Sangsiriwut K, Pooruk P, Boonnak K, Khanyok R, Thawachsupa P, Kijphati R, Sawanpanyalert P. Molecular characterization of the complete genome of human influenza H5N1 virus isolates from Thailand. J Gen Virol 2005; 86: 423-33.

4. Kneller DG, Cohen FE, Langridge R. Improvements in Protein Secondary Structure Prediction by an Enhanced Neural Network. J Mol Biol 1990; 214: 171-182.

5. Lund O, Nielsen M, Lundegaard C, Worning P. CPHmodels 2.0: X3M a Computer Program to Extract 3D Models," Abstract at the CASP5 conference A102, 2002.

6. Butler D. Alarms ring over bird flu mutations. Nature 2006; 439: 248-9.

7. Enserink M. Avian influenza. Amid mayhem in Turkey, experts see new chances for research. Science 2006; 311: 314-5.

CHAPTER 7

LEGIONELLA AND FREE LIVING AMOEBA CONTAMINATION IN NATURAL HOT SPRING POOLS IN THAILAND: OVERVIEW

Viroj Wiwanitkit[1]

[1]Wiwanitkit House, Bangkhae, Bangkok Thailand 10160

Address correspondence to: Professor Viroj Wiwanitkit, Wiwanitkit House, Bangkhae, Bangkok Thailand 10160 Email: wviroj@yahoo.com

Abstract: *Legionella* is important human pathogen.The surveillance for legionella in water reservoir is suggested. Contamination by legionella in natural hot springs may pose a significant health risk to people who use such water for recreation activities.The aim of this work is to summarize the pattern on legionella contamination in hot spring pools in Thailand. According to the search, there are 13 on radon in 83 hot spring pools in Thailand (December 2007). The number of hot springs with legionella contamination is equal to 48 (57.8 %). In addition to legionella, situation on free living amoeba in hot spring pools in Thailand is also presented in this article.

Keywords: legionella, hot spring.

1. LEGIONELLA CONTAMINATION IN HOT SPRING POOLS IN THAILAND

Introduction

Legionella is an important human pathogen. Infection with Legionella spp. is an important cause of community- and hospital-acquired pneumonia, occurring both sporadically and in outbreaks [1]. Infection with Legionella spp. ranks among the three most common causes of severe pneumonia in the community setting, and is isolated in 1-40% of cases of hospital-acquired pneumonia [1]. Legionella is an environmental pathogens that have found an ecologic niche in drinking and hot water supplies [2-3].

The surveillance for legionella in water reservoir is suggested [4]. Contamination by legionella in natural hot springs may pose a significant health risk to people who use such water for recreation activities. There are some reports on infectious cases of legionella infections due to contact to contaminated hot spring pools water [5]. To manage the water contamination by legionella is a focus in management of hot spring pools for tourist purpose. The aim of this work is to summarize the pattern on legionella contamination in hot spring pools in Thailand.

Materials and methods

Primary data

This study was designed as a descriptive retrospective study. A literature review on the performed the literature review from database of the published works cited in the Index Medicus and Science Citation Index using key word "legionella" and "hot spring".The reports that did not relate to monitoring on legionella in hot spring pools in Thailand or lacked English text or contained no complete data were excluded for further analysis.

Statistical analysis

Descriptive statistics were used in analysis. All the statistical analyses in this study were

made using SPSS 7.0 for Windows Program.

Results

According to the search there are 13 reports [6-18] on radon in 83 hot spring pools in Thailand(December 2007). The number of hot spring with legionella contamination is equal to 48 (57.8 %). There is a statistical significant correlation between setting and prevalence of legionella contamination (Table 1)

Table 1. Settings and prevalence of legionella contamination in hot spring pools in Thailand.

Settings*	Number of pools	Number of pools with legionella contamination
Northern region	27	5
Southern region	20	18
Eastern region	4	3
Western region	10	10
Central region	22	12

*There are six geographical regions in Thailand; northern, southern, eastern, western, northeastern and central regions. There is no hot spring pool in northeastern region.

Discussion

Natural mineral water has long been used worldwide for bathing and health purposes [19]. A contamination in hot spring pool is of interest [19]. Legionella contamination is noted to be an important public threaten. There are some recent reports on legionellosis outbreak due to legionella contamination in hot spring pools [6, 20]. The Hiuga City Committee directed 5 items: 1) Fix the manual for maintenance and management of the bath. 2) Keep sufficient overflow of bath water. 3) Put disinfection of filters into practice. 4) Precise measurement and control of the residual chlorine concentration in bath water. 5) Replacement of filtrating material from crushed porous ceramic into natural sand for sanitation control for legionella in ground hot spring pools [20].

At present, Thailand is famous for health spas and natural hot springs among local people and tourists.According to this work, there is a variation in the prevalence of legionella contamination in hot spring pools among different settings. This rate is similar to that of nearby Asian countries [21-22]. Focusing on the setting of the hot spring pools in this study, it seems that the hot spring pools in Western and Southern regions of Thailand are usually contaminated and implies that the hot spring in this region might not safe for direct usage.

Conclusion

There is a considerable contamination of legionella in hot spring pools in Thailand.

2. FREE LIVING AMOEBA CONTAMINATION IN HOT SPRING POOLS IN THAILAND

Free living ameba is an important human pathogen. Acanthameba keratitis caused by Acanthameba spp. and Naegleria meningoencephalitis caused by Naegleria spp. are the two most lethal free living ameba infections [23]. Contamination of free living ameba in the water reservoir is a great public health concern [23]. Free living ameba can be isolated from a variety of habitats including fresh water, thermal discharges of power plants, soil and sewage [24]. Contamination by free living ameba in natural hot springs may pose a significant health risk to people who use such water for recreation activities [25]. There are some reports on lethal cases of free living ameba infections due to contact to contaminated hot spring pools water [26-27]. To manage the water contamination by free living ameba is a focus in management of hot spring pools for tourist purpose. The aim of this work is to summarize the pattern on free living ameba in hot spring pools in Thailand.

This study was designed as a descriptive retrospective study. A literature review on the papers concerning free living ameba contamination in hot spring pools in Thailand was performed. The author performed the literature review from database of the published works cited in the Index Medicus and Science Citation Index using key word "ameba" and "hot spring". The reports that did not relate to monitoring on free living ameba contamination in hot spring pools in Thailand or lacked English text or contained no complete data were excluded for further analysis. Descriptive statistics were used in analysis. All the statistical analyses in this study were made using SPSS 7.0 for Windows Program.

According to the search there are 13 reports [6 -18] on radon in 83 hot spring pools in Thailand (December 2007). The number of hot spring with free living ameba contamination is equal to 27 (32.5 %). There is a statistical significant correlation between setting and prevalence of free living ameba contamination (Table 2).

Table 2. Settings and prevalence of free living ameba contamination in hot spring pools in Thailand.

Settings*	Number of pools	Number of pools with free living ameba contamination	
		Acanthameba spp	*Naegleria spp.*
Northern region	27	1	0
Southern region	20	14	9
Eastern region	4	0	0
Western region	10	0	0
Central region	22	12	12

*There are six geographical regions in Thailand; northern, southern, eastern, western, northeastern and central regions. There is no hot spring pool in northeastern region.

Natural mineral water has long been widely used aiming at bathing and health purposes [19]. A contamination in hot spring pool is of interest [19]. At present, Thailand is very famous and becomes the target for health spas and natural hot springs among local people and tourists. According to this work, there is a variation in the prevalence of free living ameba in hot spring pools among different settings. However, this rate is not different from those reports in other Asian and Western countries [28]. Focusing on the setting of the hot spring pools in this study, it seems that the hot spring pools in Southern and Central regions of Thailand are usually contaminated and implies that the hot spring in this region might not safe for direct usage. However, it should be noted that most of the hot springs in these two regions are not developed for tourism and the system for control of contamination should be not good.

3. REFERENCES

1.   Diederen BM. Legionella spp. and Legionnaires' disease.J Infect. 2008 Jan; 56(1): 1-12.

2.   Leclerc H, Schwartzbrod L, Dei-Cas E. Microbial agents associated with waterborne diseases.Crit Rev Microbiol. 2002; 28(4): 371-409.

3.   Seidel K. Bacteriological and hygienic aspects of a drinking and bathing water study]

4.   Schriftenr Ver Wasser Boden Lufthyg. 1985; 63: 149-57.

5.   Fujii J, Yoshida S. Legionella infection and control in occupational and environmental health.Rev Environ Health. 1998 Oct-Dec; 13(4): 179-203.

6.   Kanghae T, Pinyopornpanich S, Paveekittipornt W, Suphachaiyakit T, Tepan J, Mussakarn T, Sukthana Y, Lekkla A, Wanabongse P, Bovornkitti S. Study of natural hot springs in Southern Thailand. Intern Med J Thai. 2004 Oct -Dec; 20(4): 277-281.

7.   Kietmetha V, Jirananakhorn J, Kanghae T, Paveenkittiporn W, Wootta W, Dejsirilert S, Kruasilp J, Sukthana Y, Lekkla A, Suthikornchai C, Wanaponse P, Noomaun A, Bovornkitti S. Study of natural hot springs, Patalung and Trang Province. Intern Med J Thai. 2004 Jul-Sep; 20(3) : 207-210.

8.   Kwanmuaeng B, Wiwat L, Sulthana Y, Lekkla A, Suthikornchai C, Wootta W, Paveenkittiporn W, Dejsirilert S, Kruasilp J, Wanapongse P, Bovornkitti S. Study of Natural hot springs in Nakhon Si Thammarat and Surat Thani Provinces. 2004 Jul-Sep; 20(3): 168-173.

9.   Kruasilp J, Charanasri C, Wootta W, Wanapongse P, Bovornkitti S. Intern Med J Thai. 2004 Jan-Mar; 20(1): 43-45.

10. Lekkla A, Suthikornchai C, Sukhthana Y, Paveenkittiporn W, Wootta W, Wanabongse P, Bovornkitti S. Study of natural hot springs in central Thailand. Intern Med J Thai. 2004 Oct-Dec; 20(4): 304-307.

11. Paveenkittiporn W, Wootta W, Dejsirilert S, Harnwongsa T, Bovornkitti S. Pathogenic organisms in natural hot spring water. J Health Sci. 2004 Jan-Feb; 13(1) : 27-31

12. Pongpanitanont P, Paveenkittiporn W, Wootta W, Dejsirilert S, Kruasilp J, Sukhthana Y, Lekkla A, Suthikornchai C, Wanaponse P, Khanthanont K, Bovornkitti S. Study of hot springs in Phang-nga Province. Intern Med J Thai. 2004 Jul -Sep; 20(3): 215-217.

13. Puthimethee V, Wanapongse P, Wootta W, Paveenkittiporn W, Dejsirilert S, Sukhthana Y, Lekkla A, Suthikornchai C, Bovornkitti S. Study of natural hot springs in Kamphaengphet Provinces . Intern Med J Thai. 2004 Jul-Sep; 20,3 : 225-227.

14. Sudthikanawiwat S, Chanasit V, Paveenkittiporn W, Wootta W, Dejsirilert S, Kruasilp J, Wanapongse P, BovornkittiS. Study of natural hot springs in Eastern Thailand. Intern Med J Thai. 2004 Jul -Sep; 20(3): 165-167.

15. Tanthanasrikul S, Warahas S, Siratharanonta J, Kruasilp J, Wootta W, Wanapongse P, Bovornkitti S. Study of Natural Hot springs in western Thailand. Intern Med J Thai. 2004 Apr-Jun; 20(2): 108-111.

16. Tepant J, Mussakarn T, Kruasilp J, Wootta W, Wanapongse P, Bovornkitti S. Potential hazards in natural hot springs, Krabi Province, Thailand. Intern Med J Thai. 2004 Jan-Mar; 20(1) : 46-48.

17. Watanakul P, Paveenkittiporn P, Wootta W, Kruasilp J, Sukthana J, Lekkla A, Suthikornchai C, Wanaponse P, Bovornkitti S. Study of natural hot springs in Ranong and Chumporn Provinces. Intern Med J Thai. 2004 Jul-Sep; 20(3): 218-221.

18. Wutta W, Wanapongse P, Paweenkittiporn W, Dejsirilert S, Kruasilp J, Charanasri C, Bovornkitti S.Study of natural hot springs : Rachaburi Province. J Health Sci. 2004 Jan -Feb; 13(1): 32-36.

19. Okada M, Kawano K, Kura F, Amemura-Maekawa J, Watanabe H, Yagita K, Endo T, Suzuki S. The largest outbreak of legionellosis in Japan associated with spa baths: epidemic curve and environmental investigation. Kansenshogaku Zasshi. 2005 Jun; 79(6): 365-74.

20. Sukthana Y, Lekkla A, Sutthikornchai C, Wanapongse P, Vejjajiva A, Bovornkitti S. Spa, springs and safety.Southeast Asian J Trop Med Public Health. 2005; 36 Suppl 4: 10-6.

21. Yabuuchi E, Agata K. An outbreak of legionellosis in a new facility of hot spring bath in Hiuga City. Kansenshogaku Zasshi. 2004 Feb; 78(2): 90-8.

22. Lin YE, Lu WM, Huang HI, Huang WK. Environmental survey of Legionella pneumophila in hot springs in Taiwan. J Toxicol Environ Health A. 2007 Jan; 70(1): 84-7.

23. Schuster FL, Visvesvara GS. Free-living amoebae as opportunistic and non-opportunistic pathogens of humans and animals. Int J Parasitol. 2004 Aug; 34(9): 1001-27.

24. Visvesvara GS, Stehr-Green JK. Epidemiology of free-living ameba infections. J Protozool. 1990 Jul-Aug; 37(4): 25S-33S.

25. Lekkla A, Sutthikornchai C, Bovornkitti S, Sukthana Y. Free-living ameba contamination in natural hot springs in Thailand. Southeast Asian J Trop Med Public Health. 2005; 36 Suppl 4: 5-9.

26. Cursons R, Sleigh J, Hood D, Pullon D. A case of primary amoebic meningoencephalitis: North Island, New Zealand. N Z Med J. 2003 Dec 12; 116(1187): U712.

27. Ellis-Pegler R. Primary amoebic meningoencephalitis--rare and lethal. N Z Med J. 2003 Dec 12; 116(1187): U705.

28. Kuroki T, Yagita K, Yabuuchi E, Agata K, Ishima T, Katsube Y, Endo T. Isolation of Legionella and free-living amoebae at hot spring spas in Kanagawa, Japan. Kansenshogaku Zasshi. 1998 Oct; 72(10): 1050-5.

CHAPTER 8

ENCEPHALOPATHY IN DENGUE WITH HEPATIC FAILURE, SUMMARY OF THAI CASES

Viroj Wiwanitkit[1]

[1]*Wiwanitkit House, Bangkhae, Bangkok Thailand 10160*

Address correspondence to: Professor Viroj Wiwanitkit, Wiwanitkit House, Bangkhae, Bangkok Thailand 10160 Email: wviroj@yahoo.com

Abstract: Dengue infection is a major vector-borne disease. The classical sings and symptoms of this infection include high fever, violent headache, chill and rash. However, there are a number of atypical forms of dengue infection including those presented with severe liver dysfunction. Sporadic case reports of dengue hepatic encephalopathy are documented in Thailand. Here, the author presents a summative study on the clinical presentation and outcome among Thai patients with dengue encephalopathy in the previous studies. A literature review on the prospective studies concerning dengue hepatic encephalopathy in Thailand was performed. According to this study, 4 reports covering 19 cases (12 females and 7 males) of dengue encephalopathy among the Thai can be detected. The summative on clinical presentation of all patients are presented in Table 1. The average age (mean $\pm$ SD) of all subjects is 8.0 $\pm$ 3.0 (range = 2-13 years old). Classified by grade on dengue infection, there are 14 grade IV, 4 grade III and 1 grade II. Most of the hepatic encephalopathy occur in convalescent stage (14 cases, 73.7 %). Concerning the depth of hepatic encephalopathy, there are 8 level IV, 6 level III, 4 level II and 1 level I. Of 16 known cases, the duration of encephalopathy ranges from 0.8 to 26 days (average 8.2 $\pm$ 6.6 days). Of 15 known cases, the liver span ranges from 2 to 6 cm (average 3.7 $\pm$ 1.2 cm). Concerning the laboratory investigation, severe hepatitis (SGOT and SGPT > 200 U/L) can be seen in all cases. Hypoglycemia and hyponatremia can be detected in 6 and 5 cases, respectively. Most of the cases (15 cases, 78.9 %) received conventional treatment and most (12 cases, 63.2 %) recovered completely.

Keywords: dengue, hepatic encephalopathy.

1. INTRODUCTION

Dengue infection is a major public health problem, affecting children in the Southeast Asia Region. Up to 2-3 epidemics per year have been reported [1]. The classical form of this infection has an incubation period of 5-8 days following by the onset of fever, violent headache, chill and rash developing after 3-4 days. The fever usually lasts 4-7 days and most people had a complete recovery without any complication [2-4]. However, there are a number of atypical forms of dengue infection including those presented with severe liver dysfunction [5].

However, there are only a few reports concerning the liver dysfunction among the patients with dengue infections. A recent report of Pancharoen *et al.* revealed that average level of transaminase enzyme was higher than those who had more severe dengue infections [6]. In 2004, Chen *et al.* reported that strong correlation was found between T cell activation and hepatic cellular infiltration in immunocompetent mice infected with dengue virus [7]. They noted that the kinetics of liver enzyme elevation also correlated with that of T cell activation and suggested a relationship between T cell infiltration and elevation of liver enzymes [7]. An important complication due to severe liver dysfunction in dengue patients is hepatic encephalopathy. According to a recent study of Attavinijtrakarn in Thailand, hepatic encephalopathy is the most important complication in the dengue patients presenting with severe elevation liver enzymes [8]. Sporadic case reports of dengue hepatic encephalopathy are documented in Thailand. Here, the author presents a summative study on the clinical presentation and outcome among Thai patients with dengue encephalopathy in the previous studies.

2. MATERIALS AND METHODS

This study was designed as a descriptive retrospective study. A literature review on the prospective studies concerning case reports of dengue hepatic encephalopathy in Thailand was performed. The author performed the literature review from database of the published works cited in the Index Medicus and Science Citation Index. The author also reviewed the published works in all 256 local Thai journals, which is not included in the international citation index, for the report of dengue hepatic encephalopathy in Thailand. The clinical presentation as well as the outcome in all included reports were summarized. Descriptive statistics were used in analysis. All the statistical analyses in this study were made using SPSS 7.0 for Windows Program.

3. RESULTS

According to this study, 4 reports [8-11] covering 19 cases (12 females and 7 males) of dengue encephalopathy among the Thai can be detected. All patients have no coexistent viral hepatitis, which is also common in Thailand. The summative on clinical presentation of all patients are presented in Table 1. The average age (mean $\pm$ SD) of all subjects is 8.0 ± 3.0 (range = 2-13 years old). Classified by WHO classification on severity of dengue infection, there are 14 grade IV, 4 grade III and 1 grade II. Most of the hepatic encephalopathy occur in convalescent stage (14 cases, 73.7 %). Concerning the depth of hepatic encephalopathy [12], there are 8 level IV, 6 level III, 4 level II and 1 level I. Of 16 known cases, the duration of encephalopathy ranges from 0.8 to 26 days (average 8.2 ± 6.6 days). Of 15 known cases, the liver span ranges from 2 to 6 cm (average 3.7 ± 1.2 cm).

Concerning the laboratory investigation, severe hepatitis (SGOT and SGPT > 200 U/L) and coagulopathy (prolonged PT and PTT more than 2 times) can be seen in all cases. Hypoglycemia and hyponatremia can be detected in 6 and 5 cases, respectively. Most of the cases (15 cases, 78.9 %) received conventional treatment and most (12 cases, 63.2 %) have fully recovery. There is no significant correlation between outcome and method of treatment and hypoglycemia and hyponatremia (Chi Square test, P > 0.05).

Table 1. The summative on clinical presentation of 19 patients with dengue hepatic encephalopathy.

No	Report	Sex	Age (year)	Grade of dengue	Stage at onset*	Depth	Duration (day)	Size of liver (cm)	Treatment**
1	[8]	M	9	IV	C	I	N/A	5	C
2	[8]	F	6	IV	C	III	4	3	C
3	[8]	F	7	IV	C	III	17	3	C
4	[8]	F	11	IV	C	IV	26	4	C
5	[8]	F	7	IV	C	IV	24	4	C
6	[9]	F	10	IV	C	III	5	6	E
7	[9]	F	12	IV	C	IV	6	2	E
8	[9]	F	6	III	T	III	2	5	C
9	[9]	M	5	IV	C	II	2	5	C
10	[9]	M	4	III	C	IV	4	2	C
11	[9]	F	7	IV	T	III	1.5	3	C
12	[9]	M	7	IV	T	III	0.8	N/A	C
13	[9]	M	6	IV	C	II	1.5	4	C
14	[9]	M	8	III	C	III	6	3	C
15	[9]	F	2	IV	C	II	1.5	3	C
16	[9]	M	13	IV	T	III	0.9	N/A	C
17	[9]	F	9	III	C	II	3	N/A	E
18	[10]	F	11	IV	C	IV	N/A	N/A	E
19	[11]	F	12	II	C	IV	N/A	4	C

*C = convalescent stage, T = toxic state

**C = conventional therapy, E = exchange transfusion therapy

Table 2. The summative on important laboratory findings of 19 patients with dengue hepatic encephalopathy.

No	Report	Severe hepatitis*	Hypoglycemia	Hyponatremia	Liver pathology	Outcome**
1	[8]	Yes	No	No	N/A	Recovery
2	[8]	Yes	No	No	N/A	Recovery
3	[8]	Yes	No	No	N/A	Recovery
4	[8]	Yes	No	Yes	N/A	Death
5	[8]	Yes	No	Yes	N/A	Death
6	[9]	Yes	No	No	Fatty change	Recovery
7	[9]	Yes	No	No	N/A	Recovery
8	[9]	Yes	No	Yes	N/A	Recovery
9	[9]	Yes	No	No	N/A	Recovery
10	[9]	Yes	Yes	No	N/A	Recovery
11	[9]	Yes	Yes	No	N/A	Death
12	[9]	Yes	No	Yes	Focal hemorrhage	Death
13	[9]	Yes	Yes	No	Focal necrosis	Death
14	[9]	Yes	Yes	No	N/A	Death
15	[9]	Yes	Yes	No	N/A	Recovery
16	[9]	Yes	Yes	Yes	N/A	Death
17	[9]	Yes	No	No	Fatty change	Recovery
18	[10]	Yes	No	No	N/A	Recovery
19	[11]	Yes	No	No	N/A	Recovery

*Severe hepatitis is determined when ALT and AST > 200 U/L

** The cause of death in all fatal cases is severe gastrointestinal bleeding and renal failure

4. DISCUSSION

Although liver is not the target organ of dengue virus, several liver pathological findings including fatty change, centrilobular necrosis, and monocyte infiltration in the portal tract, are reported in previously published literature [5]. Concerning the encephalopathy among the patients with dengue infection, most are due to hypoxia corresponding to shock [13]. An encephalopathy due to hepatic cause is an extremely rare presentation. The author hereby reports the summarization of the clinical presentation of 19 Thai cases with dengue hepatic encephalopathy.

The findings from this study are similar to a recent report on 8 cases of dengue hepatic encephalopathy in Malaysia [14]. The episodes are usually more common in the patients with severe dengue infection (grade III and grade IV) [14]. Most of the cases start at convalescent stage. Indeed, the increase antibody in the convalescent stage might be a contributing factor to hepatic encephalopathy in dengue infection [15].

Concerning the fatality rate, the rate in this study (36.8 %) is higher than the previous report by Lum *et al.* (about 16.7 %) [14]. Considering the death cases, the gastrointestinal bleeding and acute renal failure is the common cause. The author hereby can demonstrate that either conventional treatment by fluid supportive, symptomatic as well as prevention of bleeding complications, can provide similar outcome to exchange transfusion therapy.

5. REFERENCES

1.   Thisyakorn U, Thisyakorn C. Diseases caused by arboviruses-dengue hemorrhagic fever and Japanese B encephalitits. Med J Aus 1994; 160: 22-6.

2.   Guzman MG, Kouri G. Dengue: an update. Lancet Infect Dis. 2002; 2: 33-42.

3.   da Fonseca BA, Fonseca SN. Dengue virus infections. Curr Opin Pediatr 2002; 14: 67-71.

4.   Solomon T, Mallewa M. Dengue and other emerging flaviviruses. J Infect. 2001; 42: 104-15.

5.   Huerre MR, Lan NT, Marianneau P, Hue NB, Khun H, Hung NT, Khen NT, Drouet MT, Huong VT, Ha DQ, Buisson Y, Deubel V. Liver histopathology and biological correlates in five cases of fatal dengue fever in Vietnamese children. Virchows Arch 2001; 438: 107-15 .

6.   Pancharoen C, Rungsarannont A, Thisyakorn U. Hepatic dysfunction in dengue patients with various severity. J Med Assoc Thai 2002; 85 (Suppl 1): S298-S301.

7.   Chen HC, Lai SY, Sung JM, Lee SH, Lin YC, Wang WK, Chen YC, Kao CL, King CC, Wu-Hsieh BA. Lymphocyte activation and hepatic cellular infiltration in immunocompetent mice infected by dengue virus. J Med Virol 2004; 73: 419-31.

8.   Attavinijtrakarn P. Hepatic dysfunction in dengue hemorrhagic fever in Paholpolpayuhasaena Hospital. Thai J Pediatr 2000; 39: 265-276.

9.   Pongrithsukda V, Chunharas A. Dengue hemorrhagic fever and hepatic encephalopathy. Ramathibodi Med J 1986; 9: 11-18.

10.   Pamonsut S. Dengue hemorrhagic fever with liver failure and encephalopathy in Thabsakae Hospital: Case study. Office Commun Dis Control Reg 1 J M 2003 ; 7: 82-85.

11.   Sirivichayakul C, Sabcharoen A, Chanthavanich P, Pengsaa K, Chokejindachai W, Prarinyanupharb V. Dengue infection with unusual manifestations: a case report. J Med Assoc Thai 2000; 83: 325-9.

12.   Rogers JB Jr. Neurologic complications of gastrointestinal tract diseases. N Y State J Med 1973; 73: 971-6.

13.   Vasanawathana S. Encephalopathy in DHF in Khon Kaen Hospital. Khon Kaen Med J 1992; 16: 91-104.

14.   Lum LC, Lam SK, George R, Devi S. Fulminant hepatitis in dengue infection. Southeast Asian J Trop Med Public Health 1993; 24: 467-71.

15.   Lei HY, Yeh TM, Liu HS, Lin YS, Chen SH, Liu CC. Immunopathogenesis of dengue virus infection. J Biomed Sci 2001; 8: 377-88.

CHAPTER 9

PREVALENCE OF CRYPTOSPORIDIOSIS AMONG THAI HIV-INFECTED PATIENTS WITH DIARRHEA AT PRESENT AND IN THE PAST DECADE: IS THERE ANY EFFECT OF HAART THERAPY

Viroj Wiwanitkit[1]

[1]*Wiwanitkit House, Bangkhae, Bangkok Thailand 10160*

Address correspondence to: Professor Viroj Wiwanitkit, Wiwanitkit House, Bangkhae, Bangkok Thailand 10160 Email: wviroj@yahoo.com

Abstract: An important parasitic infection among HIV infected patients is the cryptosporidiosis. *Cryptosporidium parvum* is an intestinal parasitic protozoon that causes severe diarrhea and may lead to death in immunocompromised hosts. In HIV infected cases with cryptosporidiasis, four main clinical syndromes were identified: chronic diarrhea, choleralike disease, transient diarrhea, and relapsing illness. In this paper, the authors presented the prevalence of cryptosporidiosis among Thai HIV-infected patients with diarrhea in comparison to the previous noted prevalence in the past decade. The prevalence of among Thai HIV infected patients with diarrhea in the previous decade is equal to 7.14 %. The present prevalence of among Thai HIV infected patients with diarrhea is investigated with the same protocol. Overall 25 HIV infected cases could be detected giving the prevalence equal to 18.95 % (25/193). Of interest, although the HAART therapy is easily available in Thailand, at present the prevalence of cryptosporidiosis is still very high in the HIV seropositive patients with diarrhea. Therefore, the authors hereby propose that the wide distribution of HAART therapy did not affect the prevalence of cyrptosporidiosis among HIV seropositive patients with diarrhea.

Keywords: HIV, cryptosporidiosis, HAART therapy.

1. INTRODUCTION

One of the major health problems among HIV seropositive patients is superimposed infection due to the defect of immunity [1]. Furthermore, intestinal parasite infection, which is also one of the basic health problems in tropical region, is common in these patients. In Thailand, a tropical country in Southeast Asia, HIV infection is a major problem, like in other regional countries. It has been estimated that a million people are infected with HIV infection in Thailand [2]. And it also the possibly higher undetected HIV infection in the community.

An important parasitic infection among HIV infected patients is the cryptosporidiosis. Cryptosporidium parvum is an intestinal parasitic protozoa that causes severe diarrhea and may lead to death in immunocompromised hosts. In developing regions of the world, Cryptosporidium constitute part of the complex group of parasitic, bacterial and viral diseases that impair the ability to achieve full potential and impair development and socio-economic improvements [3]. It has been included in list of WHO Neglected Diseases Initiative since 2004 [3]. In medicine, cryptosporidiosis is very common in patients with HIV/AIDS and remains a treat to public health [4-6]. In HIV infected cases with cryptosporidiasis, four main clinical syndromes were identified: chronic diarrhea, choleralike disease, transient diarrhea, and relapsing illness [4-6]. In this paper, the authors presented the prevalence of cryptosporidiosis among Thai HIV-infected patients with diarrhea at present with comparison to the previous noted prevalence in a past decade.

2. MATERIALS AND METHODS

Protocol for evaluation of cryptosporidosis among Thai HIV infected patients with diarrhea are shown below

- Subjects and operative definition for diarrhea and HIV infection

A total of 193 subjects were enrolled into this study. At each clinic visits, patients were asked whether they have any diarrhea or not. If so they were asked to participate in the study. The inclusion criteria is having diarrhea, history of unformed stool for at least 1 day. All subjects in this study were known cases of HIV/AIDS. All received HAART therapy. Exclusion was set in any cases without agreement to give consent for the study.

- Laboratory analysis

Fresh stool specimens were collected in plastic containers approximiately 10 gms and processed within 24 hrs, and the specimens were examined for intestinal parasites by direct examination, formol ethyl-acetate concentration technique, and modified Ziehl-Neelsen stain under light microscope. The stool specimens were performed at the standard clinical microscopy laboratory. If stool examination could not be done, the specimen should be kept in box with ice packs or in the refrigerator (4°C) until processing.

- Ethical approval

The study was approved by the Ethical Committee on Research Involving Human Subject of Faculty of Medicine of the university and Rajavithi Hospital, Ministry of Public Health, Bangkok. Informed consents were obtained from all patients who were over 20 years of age. This protocol is similarly applied for the previous [1] and present investigation.

3. RESULTS

Comparison between the subjects in the present and previous stuidy

The sample size in the present work is calculated based on the previous work. The sample size is the present work is sufficient to answer the question on the prevalence. The subjects in the present study were included with the same criteria as that of the previous study. The subjects were from the same socioeconomic backgroup and age group (20 to 65 years). The sex ditribution in the present work (male 65.0 %, female 35.0 %) is not is not statistically difference from that of the previous work (male 63.3 %, female 36.7 %) (proportional Z test, $p < 0.05$). The distribution of CD4+ count of the subjects in the present work (24.5 +/- 95.5 μL) is not statistically difference from that of the previous work (36.6 +/- 103.5 μL) (Unpaired T test, $p < 0.05$).

Prevalence of the cryptosporidiosis among Thai HIV infected patients in the previous decade (1998)

The prevalence of among Thai HIV infected patients with diarrhea in the previous decade is quoted from the previous report by Wiwanitkit [1]. According to this study, the prevalence of cryptosporidiosis is equal to 7.14 % (2/28).

Prevalence of the cryptosporidiosis among HIV infected patients at present (2007)

The present prevalence of among Thai HIV infected patients with diarrhea is investigated with the same protocol. Overall 25 HIV infected cases could be detected giving the prevalence equal to 18.95 % (25/193).

4. DISCUSSION

Cryptosporidiosis is a self-limited diarrheal disease that occurs in the community setting but can be chronic and potentially serious in immunocompromised patients [7]. Cryptosporidium parvum is an important emerging pathogen and a cause of severe, life-threatening disease in patients with AIDS [8]. Patients with human immunodeficiency virus infection should be made more aware of the many ways that Cryptosporidium species are transmitted, and they should be given guidance on how to reduce the risk of exposure [8]. For history of diarrhea, many studies noted a significant correlation between diarrhea and cryptosporidiosis [9-11].

It is noted that HAART might directly exert an inhibitory effect on C. parvum and the extent of this effect depended on the specific dose and the duration of treatment [12]. In this work, the authors studied the prevalence of cryptosporidiosis in HIV infected patients with diarrhea. A comparison to the previous noted prevalence, when highly active antiretroviral therapy (HAART) therapy was not available in Thailand, is also shown. The comparison was made on the two groups with similar socioeconomic background, age group, sex distribution as well as underlying CD4+ count. Of interest, although the HAART therapy is easily available in Thailand at present the prevalence of cryptosporidiosis is still very high in the HIV seropositive patients with diarrhea. Therefore, the authors hereby propose that the widely distribution of HAART therapy might not affect the prevalence of cyrptosporidiosis among HIV seropositive patients with diarrhea. However, it should be awared that HAART control on cryptosporidiosis in immunodeficient patients is not direct but might through increasing CD4-T cell counts.

5. ADDITIONAL NOTE ON DECLINDED OF PREVALENCE OF INTESTINAL HELMINTHIASIS AMONG THAI HIV-INFECTED PATIENTS WITH DIARRHEA: POSSIBLE EFFECT OF HAART THERAPY

<u>Introduction</u>

One of the major health problems among HIV seropositive patients is superimposed infection due to the defect of immunity [1]. Furthermore, intestinal parasite infection, which is also one of the basic health problems in tropical region, is common in these patients. In Thailand, a tropical country in Southeast Asia, HIV infection is a major problem, like in other regional countries. It has been estimated that a million people are infected with HIV infection in Thailand [2]. And it also the possibly higher undetected HIV infection in the community. helminth infections play a major role in the pathogenesis of HIV-1 infection in Africa and other developing areas, due to their profound effects on the host immune system, which make those infected more susceptible to HIV-1 infection and less able to cope with it [13]. Chronic immune activation with a dominant Th2 profile, and anergy, are the hallmarks of chronic helminth infection, and may therefore account for most of these effects [13]. Available epidemiological data regarding interactions between helminths and HIV are largely observational; results are variable and generally inconclusive [14]. Silva *et al.* noted that diagnosing intestinal parasites in HIV/AIDS patients is necessary [14].

Here, the authors presented the prevalence of intestinal helminthiasis among Thai HIV-infected patients with diarrhea at present with comparison to the previous note prevalence in a past decade.

<u>Materials and methods</u>

- Subjects and operative definition for diarrhea and HIV infection

A total of 193 subjects were enrolled into this study. At each clinic visits, patients were asked whether they have any diarrhea or not. If so they were asked to participate in the study. The inclusion criteria is having diarrhea, history of unformed stool for at least 1 day. All subjects in this study were known cases of HIV/AIDS. All received HAART therapy. Exclusion was set in any cases without agreement to give consent for the study.

- Laboratory analysis

Fresh stool specimens were collected in plastic containers approximiately 10 gms and processed within 24 hrs, and the specimens were examined for intestinal parasites by direct examination, formol ethyl-acetate concentration technique, and modified Ziehl-Neelsen stain under light microscope. The stool specimens were performed at the standard clinical microscopy If stool examination could not be done, the specimen should be kept in box with ice packs or in the refrigerator until processing

- Ethical approval

The study was approved by the Ethical Committee on Research Involving Human Subject of Faculty of Medicine of the university and Rajavithi Hospital, Ministry of Public Health,

Bangkok. Informed consents were obtained from all patients who were over 20 years of This protocol is similarly applied for the previous [1] and present investigation. The sample size in the present work is calculated based on the previous work.

Results

The sample size is the present work is sufficient to answer the question on the prevalence. The subjects in the present study were included with the same criteria as that of the previous study. The subjects were from the same socioeconomic backgroup and age group (20 to 65 years). The sex ditribution in the present work (male 65.0 %, female 35.0 %) is not is not statistically difference from that of the previous work (male 63.3 %, female 36.7 %) (proportional Z test, $p > 0.05$). The distribution of CD4+ count of the subjects in the present work (24.5 +/- 95.5 μL) is not statistically difference from that of the previous work (36.6 +/- 103.5 μL) (Unpaired T test, $p > 0.05$). Prevalence of the cryptosporidiosis among Thai HIV infected patients in the previous decade (1998)\par The prevalence of among Thai HIV infected patients with diarrhea in the previous decade is quoted from the previous report by Wiwanitkit [6]. According to this study, the prevalence of intestinal helminthiasis is equal to 40 % The present prevalence of among Thai HIV infected patients with diarrhea is investigated with the same protocol. Overall 25 HIV infected cases could be detected giving the prevalence equal to 0 % (0/193).

Discussion

Intestinal helminthiasis is an important gastrointestinal problem all around the world especially the underdeveloped and tropical countries. Mohandas *et al.* noted that 75% of HIV infected patients with intestinal helminthasis had diarrhea [15]. Therefore, searching for intestinal helminthic infestation is recommended for the HIV infected cases presenting with diarrhea [1, 15-16]. In HIV infected patients, the prevalence of intestinal helminthais is very high in the patients who are not prescribed for HAART [5-6]. However, the report on the epidemiology in the setting with HAART has never been set.

In this work, the authors studied the prevalence of intestinal helminthiasis in HIV infected patients with diarrhea. A comparison to the previous note prevalence, when highly active antiretroviral therapy (HAART) therapy was not available in Thailand, is also shown. The comparison was made on the two groups with similar socioeconomic background, age group, sex distribution as well as underlying CD4+ count. Of interest, the HAART therapy is easily available in Thailand at present and the prevalence of intestinal helminthiasis is significantly decreased in the HIV seropositive patients with diarrhea. Therefore, the authors hereby propose that the widely distribution of HAART therapy strongly affect the prevalence of intestinal heminthiasis among HIV seropositive patients with diarrhea. In addition, the author suggested searching for the other corresponding causes for diarrhea in HIV-infected patients including opportunistic intestinal protozoa enterovirus are necessary for finding the exact etiology.

Conclusion

One of the major health problems among HIV seropositive patients is superimposed infection due to the defect of immunity. Furthermore, intestinal helminthiasis, which is also one of the basic health problems in tropical region, is common in these patients. In this paper, the authors presented the prevalence of intestinal helminthasis among Thai HIV-infected patients with diarrhea at present with comparison to the previous noted prevalence in a past decade.Of interest, the HAART therapy is easily available in Thailand at present and the prevalence of intestinal helminthiasis is significantly decreased in the HIV seropositive patients with diarrhea. Therefore, the authors hereby propose that the widely distribution of HAART therapy strongly affect the prevalence of intestinal heminthiasis among HIV seropositive patients with diarrhea. In addition, the author suggested searching for the other corresponding causes for diarrhea in HIV-infected patients including opportunistic intestinal protozoa enterovirus are necessary.

6. ACKNOLEDGEMENT

The author hereby would like to acknowledge Associate Professor Mayuna Srisupanant who gives the data for comparative study in this work.

7. REFEERENCES

1.   Wiwanitkit V. Intestinal parasite infestation in HIV infected patients.Curr HIV Res 2006; 4: 87-96.

2.   Surasiengsunk S, Kiranandana S, Wongboonsin K, Garnett GP, Anderson RM, van Griensven GJ. Demographic impact of the HIV epidemic in Thailand. AIDS 1998, 12: 775-784.

3.   Savioli L, Smith H, Thompson A. Giardia and Cryptosporidium join the 'Neglected Diseases Initiative'. Trends Parasitol 2006; 22: 203-8.

4.   Chappell CL, Okhuysen PC. Cryptosporidiosis. Curr Opin Infect Dis 2002; 15: 523-7.

5.   Dionisio D. Cryptosporidiosis in HIV-infected patients. J Postgrad Med 2002; 48: 215- 6.

6.   Manabe YC, Clark DP, Moore RD, Lumadue JA, Dahlman HR, Belitsos PC, Chaisson RE, Sears CL. Cryptosporidiosis in patients with AIDS: correlates of disease and survival. Clin Infect Dis 1998; 27: 536-42.

7.   Chappell CL, Okhuysen PC. Cryptosporidiosis. Curr Opin Infect Dis 2002; 15: 523-7.

8.   Juranek DD. Cryptosporidiosis: sources of infection and guidelines for prevention. Clin Infect Dis 1995; 21 Suppl 1: S57-61.

9.   Cornet M, Romand S, Warszawski J, Bouree P. Factors associated with microsporidial and cryptosporidial diarrhea in HIV infected patients. Parasite 1996; 3: 397-401.

10.   Tadesse A, Kassu A. Intestinal parasite isolates in AIDS patients with chronic diarrhea in Gondar Teaching Hospital, North west Ethiopia. Ethiop Med J 2005; 43: 93-6.

11.   Lopez-Velez R, Tarazona R, Garcia Camacho A, Gomez-Mampaso E, Guerrero A, Moreira V, Villanueva R. Intestinal and extraintestinal cryptosporidiosis in AIDS patients. Eur J Clin Microbiol Infect Dis 1995; 14: 677-81.

12.   Morales Gomez MA. Highly Active AntiRetroviral Therapy and cryptosporidiosis. Parassitologia 2004 Jun; 46(1-2): 95-9.

13.   Borkow G, Bentwich Z. HIV and helminth co-infection: is deworming necessary? Parasite Immunol. Helminths and HIV infection: epidemiological observations on immunological hypotheses. Parasite Immunol 2006 Nov; 28: 613-23.

14.   Silva CV, Ferreira MS, Borges AS, Costa-Cruz JM. Intestinal parasitic infections in HIV/AIDS patients: experience at a teaching hospital in central Brazil. Scand J Infect Dis 2005; 37: 211-5.

15.   Mohandas, Sehgal R, Sud A, Malla N. Prevalence of intestinal parasitic pathogens in HIV-seropositive individuals in Northern India. Jpn J Infect Dis 2002 Jun; 55(3): 83-4.

16.   Tadesse A, Kassu A. Intestinal parasite isolates in AIDS patients with chronic diarrhea in Gondar Teaching Hospital, North west Ethiopia. Ethiop Med J 2005; 43: 93-6.

CHAPTER 10

CAPILLARIA PHILLIPINENSIS INFECTION, SUMMARY FROM 12 PREVIOUSLY NOTES THAI CASES

Pongsatorn Kue-A-Pai[1] and Viroj Wiwanitkit[2]

1Faculty of Medicine Siriraj Hospital, Mahidol University, Chulalongkorn University, Bangkok 10330 Thailand;

2 Wiwanitkit House, Bangkhae, Bangkok Thailand 10160

Address correspondence to: Professor Viroj Wiwanitkit, Wiwanitkit House, Bangkhae, Bangkok Thailand 10160 Email: wviroj@yahoo.com

Abstract: CONTEXT: *Capillaria philippinensis* infection is a round worm infection. Capillariasis philippinensis is considered a zoonotic disease of migratory fish-eating birds.

OBJECTIVE: Here, the author performed a literature review on the reports of *C. philippinensis* in Thailand in order to summarize the characteristics of this infection among the Thai patients.

DESIGN: This study was designed as a descriptive retrospective study. A literature review of the papers concerning *C. philippinensis* infections in Thailand was performed.

RESULTS: Due to this study, there have been at least 8 reports of *C. philippinensis* infection, of which 1 case was lethal (Table 1). There are at least 12 Thai cases with *C. philippinensis* infections. The age ranges from 13 to 58 years. Of seven well-documented cases, 5 were males and 2 were females. Most (10/12) cases were detected from stool examination: One was detected by Gastroduodenoscopy: The other case (1/12) was detected after the patient died.

CONCLUSION: In conclusion, *C. philippinensis* infection is sporadically noted in Thailand. The diagnosis is usually by stool examination. The survival rate of these infections is high if the diagnosis is correct and is quite low if the diagnosis is too late. The treatment of this infection is an antiparasitic drug such as mebendazole and albendazole.

Keywords: Thai, Capillaria philippinensis infection.

1. INTRODUCTION

The nematode (roundworm) *Capillaria philippinensis* is the causative agent of human intestinal capillariasis. It was first discovered in the Philippines in 1963. The life cycle involves freshwater fish as intermediate hosts and fish-eating birds as definitive hosts. Embryonated eggs from feces fed to fish hatch and grow as larvae in the fish intestines. Infective larvae fed to fish-eating birds develop into adults. Larvae become adults in 10 to 11 days, and the first-generation females produce larvae. These larvae develop into males and egg-producing female worms. Eggs pass with the feces, reach water, embryonate, and infect fish. Autoinfection is part of the life cycle and causes hyperinfection. Humans are infected by eating small freshwater fish raw. The parasite multiplies, and symptoms of diarrhea, borborygmus, abdominal pain, and edema develop. Chronic infections lead to malnutrition, malabsorption and hence to protein and electrolyte loss, and death results from irreversible effects of the infection.

In Thailand, the first case report of C. *philippinensis* infection has been published since 1981 by Kunaratanapruk S [1-9]. Since the first case report, there have been sporadic case reports of the *C. philippinensis* in Thailand. Here, the author performed a literature review on the reports of *C. philippinensis* infections in Thailand in order to summarize the characteristics of this infection among the Thai patients.

2. MATERIALS AND METHODS

This study was designed as a descriptive retrospective study. A literature review on the papers concerning Capillaria philippinensis infection in Thailand was performed. The author performed the literature review *C. philippinensis* infection reports in Thailand from database of the published works cited in the Index Medicus and Pubmed. The author also reviewed the published works in all 256 local Thai journals, which is not included in the international citation index, for the report of infections in Thailand. The literature review was focused till March 2004.

The inclusion criteria are the literatures as case report of sporadic episode of capillariasis. The exclusion criteria are the literatures with incomplete data for further analysis. According to the literature review, reports were recruited for further study. The details of clinical presentations of the patients (such as clinical manifestation, diagnosis, treatment and discharge status) in all included reports were studied. The demographic data of all cases including age, sex and address were reviewed as well. Descriptive statistics were used in analyzing the patient characteristics and laboratory parameters for each group. All the statistical analyses in this study were made using SPSS 7.0 for Windows Program.

Table 1. Summarization on the cases of patients with capillariasis included into this study.

No	Authors	Age (years)	Sex	Address *	Diagnosis	Presentation	Treatment	Outcome
1	Pathnacharoen *et al.*, 1983 [1]	N/A	N/A	NE	Stool examination	Protein-calorie malnutrition	mebendazole 400 mg/day	Cure
2	Pathnacharoen *et al.*, 1983 [1]	N/A	N/A	NE	Stool examination	Chronic diarrhea with shock	mebendazole 400 mg/day	Cure
3	Pathnacharoen *et al.*, 1983 [1]	N/A	N/A	NE	Stool examination	Chronic diarrhea with shock	mebendazole 400 mg/day	Cure
4	Tiensripojamarn *et al.*, 1982 [2]	N/A	N/A	C	Stool examination	Chronic diarrhea with malabsorption	mebendazole 400 mg/day	Cure
5	Tiensripojamarn *et al.*, 1982 [2]	N/A	N/A	C	Stool examination	Chronic diarrhea with malabsorption	mebendazole 400 mg/day	Cure
6	Tesana *et al.*, 1983 [3]	25	Female	NE	Autopsy	Abdominal pain and borborygmi	No	Death
7	Chayakul *et al.*, 1988 [4]	58	Male	NE	Stool examination	Chronic diarrhea	mebendazole 400 mg/day	Cure
8	Chayakul *et al.*, 1988 [4]	30	Female	NE	Stool examination	Repeated diarrhea and edema	mebendazole 400 mg/day	Cure
9	Chitchang *et al.*, 1979 [5]	32	Male	C	Stool examination	Attacks of edema and diarrhea	mebendazole 400 mg/day	Cure
10	Muangmanee *et al.*, 1977[6]	47	Male	NE	Stool examination	6-month history of diarrhea and debility	mebendazole 400 mg/day	Cure
11	Thomnakarn *et al.*, 1998 [7]	52	Male	NE	Stool examination	abdominal pain, chronic diarrhea, malaise	200 mg. of Albendazole	Cure
12	Wongsawasdi *et al.*, 2002 [8]	13	Male	C	Gastroduo-de-noscopy	10-month history of chronic abdominal pain and diarrhea	mebendazole 400 mg/day	Cure

*address is classified according to the Region of Thailand; NE = Northeastern, C = Central

3. RESULTS

Due to this study, there have been at least 8 reports of *C. philippinensis* infection, of which 1 case was lethal (Table 1). There are at least 12 Thai cases with *C. philippinensis* infections. The age ranges from 13 to 58 years. Of seven well-documented cases, 5 were males and 2 were females. Most (10/12) cases were detected from stool examination: One was detected by Gastroduodenoscopy: The other case (1/12) was detected after the patient was dead. Most (11/12) cases had either chronic diarrhea or repeated diarrhea. The antiparasitic drugs were prescribed in most cases Mebendazole in 10 cases and Albendazole in 1 case.

4. DISCUSSION

C. philippinensis infection is nematode infection occurs most in the Philippines and Thailand. Human acquires *C. philippinensis* by eating of raw or uncooked fish which has infective larvae. The parasite was originally discovered in human in the Philippines but since there has also been noted in human in Thailand. *C. philippinensis* is then considered a zoonotic disorder of migratory fish-eating birds. The eggs are disseminated along flyways and infect the fish, and when fish are eaten raw, this specific medical disorder develops.

According to this series, most patients had diarrhea, abdominal pain, and edema. Few cases had malnutrition, protein-calorie malnutrition. There is an interesting death case. The treatment of this case was electrolyte Glucose and Sohamin-G replacement. After one day of treatment the patient was dead due to failure of diagnosis. After the autopsy, every stage of *C. philippinensis* was found in the patient's intestine except for its egg

Looking in the 11 cases, who received the antiparasitic treatment, the succeed can be derived by either mebendazole 400 mg daily for one month or 200 mg albendazole daily for 2 months. Conclusively, *C. philippinensis* infection is sporadically observed in Thailand. The diagnosis is usually by stool microscopic examination. The survival rate of these infections is high if the diagnosis is correct and is quite unfavorable low if the diagnosis is too late. The treatment of this infection is an antiparasitic drug such as mebendazole and albendazole.

5. REFERENCES

1.   Pathnacharoen S, Tansuphaswadikul S, Manutstitt S, Thanangkul B. Intestinal capillariasis Ramathibodi Med J 1983; 6: 277-83.

2.   Tiensripojamarn A, Jarajinda S, Veerakula K, Rutapichairuxa N. R Thai Air Force Med Gaz1982; 28: 193-7.

3.   Tesana S, Bhuripanyo K, Sanpitak P, Sithithaworn P. Intestinal capillariasis from Udon Thani Province, Northeastern part of Thailand. J Med Assoc Thai 1983; 66: 128-31.

4.   Chayakul P, Ovartlarnporn B, Kulwichit P, Piratvisut T, Kunasakdakun A. Intestinal capillariasis. J Infect Dis Antimicrob Agents 1988; 5: 187-90.

5.   Chitchang S, Chitprasong T, JanTong T, Suksala N. Intestinal capillariasis from Lopburi Province. R Thai Army Med J 1979; 32: 163-5.

6.   Muangmanee L, Aswapokee N, Vanasin B. Intestinal capillariasis. Siriraj Hosp Gaz 1977; 29: 439-45.

7.   Thomnakarn K, Penpinich C, Saietang S. Intestinal capillariasis at Khon Kaen Regional Hospital. Khon Kaen Hosp Med J 1998; 22: 65-7.

8.   Wongsawasdi L, Ukarapol N, Lertprasertsuk N. The endoscopic diagnosis of intestinal capillariasis in a child. Southeast Asian J Trop Med Public Health. 2002 Dec; 33(4): 730-2.

9.   Kunaratanapruk S, Iam-Ong S, Chatsirimongkol C. Intestinal capillariasis. Ramathibodi Med J 1981; 4: 206-13.

CHAPTER 11

OVERVIEW OF ZYGOMYCOSIS IN THAILAND

Nutchya Khemnark[1], Saranya Ngamrassamiwong[1] and Viroj Wiwanitkit[2]

[1]Faculty of Medicine, Chulalongkorn University, Bangkok Thailand 10330

[2]Wiwanitkit House, Bangkhae, Bangkok Thailand 10160

Address correspondence to: Professor Viroj Wiwanitkit, Wiwanitkit House, Bangkhae, Bangkok Thailand 10160 Email: wviroj@yahoo.com

Abstract: *Zygomycosis* is a rare fungal infection. It is noted sporadically throughout the world. In Thailand, this illness has been noted since 1978. We hereby present a retrospective study concerning the previous literatures regarding Zygomycosis in Thailand. According to this study, 27 cases of Zygomycosis of 15 literatures were studied retrospectively. Of these 27 cases, 16 were females and 11 were males. The average age was 38.5 + 18.1 years. In this study, 23 patients (85.2%) were infected with Mucorales and 4 patients were infected with Entomophthorales. Of the 23 cases with Mucorales infections, 16 patients (59.2%) were rhinocerebral, 3 patients (11.1%) were pulmonary, 3 patients (11.1%) were cutaneous and 1 patient (3.7%) was gastrointestinal. Of these 23 patients, 52.2% had DM, 17.4% had CRF, 17.4% had the history of non-steroid immunosuppressive drug use, 4.3% had the history of steroid use and 4.3% had prolonged antibiotic drug use. Of 13 Mucorales-the cases infected with adequate data for further analysis, 9 (69.2%) died. Concerning the left 4 patients (14.8%) with Entomophthorales infecions all had subcutaneous zygomycosis. None of these 4 cases died. In conclusion, the zygomycosis in Thai patients is similar to the prior reports. Nevertheless, However, we find a trend of female adult premodinance of infection.

Keywords: Mucormycosis, Thailand.

1. INTRODUCTION

Zygomycosis is an opportunistic fungal infection from the fungus in class Phycomycetes or Zygomycetes [1-16]. Medically, this disease is generated by specific fungi in the two orders: Mucorales and Entomophthorales The first group fungi includes the fungi in the genus Rhizopus, Mucor and Absidia [9]. The second one can be classified into two genuses: Basidiobolae and Conidiobolae. Generally, mucormycosis can manifest five difference forms: rhinocerebral form, pulmonary form, gastrointestinal form, cutaneous form and the disseminated form [10], which are all caused by mucorale [11]. However, there is another distinguish form, caused by Entomophthorale; the subcutaneous form [11].

Microbiologically, these fungal organisms can be found in the soil, rotten fruit [9], small bowel of amphibian and reptile [11] and decaying organic material. Concerning Mucorales, the organisms infect compromised hosts, particularly in cases of diabetic with acidosis, leukemia, lymphoma, using steroid drug, depressed immunity treatment [9] and chronic renal failure [11]. The clinical feature depends on the system and area that they infect. In contrast, Entomophthorales gradually infect tissue and nearly all patients can survive [11].

Nevertheless, both infections bring health problems in tropical countries especially in South Africa. In Thailand, there are sporadic cases of these infections [15-16]. The first report in Thailand was described by Piyarat P in 1961 [15] while the first world noted was by Paultauf in 1885 [1]. This review was made up to aware and analyze the information of zygomycosis in Thailand. According to our study, it can be said that zygomycosis is a curable disease, especially in case with early diagnosis and prompt treatment and Entomophthoromycosis show better prognosis than mycormycosis.

2. MATERIALS AND METHODS

This study was designed as a retrospective case summary to accumulate the previous reports on the literatures concerning Thai cases with Zygomycosis. Actually, it is an added up to previously publication on mucorales infection among the Thai with diabetes mellitus [17]. The data collection was performed by literature search using Pubmed and Thai Index Medicus. Those reports that have no clear definite diagnosis of Zygomycosis were excluded. The data from each literature was extracted for sex, age, address, clinical manifestation, the duration before the admission, complication, underlying cause, laboratory investigations and the result of the treatment. Then all data was analyzed using descriptive statistics. Excel for Windows Program was used for statistical calculation.

3. RESULTS

From literature searching, we could gain data of 27 Thai patients with Zygomycosis from 15 reports. There were 16 females and 11 males. Their average age was 38.5 + 18.1 years. The summarization of patient's characteristics for each case was presented in Table 1.

Table 1. The summarization of patient's characteristics for each case

Authors	Sex	Age	PTA	Type	Underlying cause	Result
Puangpornsri *et al.*, 1987 [10]	M	40 yrs	7 days	rhinocerebral	renal insufficiency	cured
Chandrakul and Sakolphadungkhet, 1961 [3]	M	52 yrs	no data	cutaneous	no data	died
Chandrakul and Sakolphadungkhet, 1961 [3]	F	33 yrs	8 days	cutaneous	no data	cured
Nutprayun *et al.*, 1979 [7]	F	21 yrs	2 wks	pulmonary	depressed immunity drug	died
Cutchavaree *et al.*, 1978 [4]	F	13 yrs	4 days	rhinocerebral	no data	died
Chandrakul and Sakolphadungkhet, 1961 [3]	F	3 mos	7 days	rhinocerebral	antibiotic drug	died
Wiriyasatiankun and Komolsuradej, 1992 [16]	F	29 yrs	3 days	rhinocerebral	DM	died
Wiriyasatiankun and Komolsuradej, 1992 [16]	F	32 yrs	2 days	rhinocerebral	DM,renal tubular acidosis	died
Prakitrittranon, 1992 [8]	F	54 yrs	3 yrs	sucutaneous	no data	cured
Aikvanich and Niampradit, 1990 [2]	F	24 yrs	4 days	rhinocerebral	depressed immunity drug	cured
Aikvanich and Niampradit, 1990 [2]	M	59 yrs	3 wks	rhinocerebral	DM,steroid drug	died
Ponglertnapagorn *et al.*, 1994 [9]	M	45 yrs	3 days	pulmonary	DM	no data
Srisukwattana *et al.*, 1986 [12]	M	5 mos	2 wks	rhinocerebral	no data	died
Luxananant, 1996 [6]	M	48 yrs	4-5 mos	gastrointestinal	no data	no data
Supasin and Supaporn, 1999 [14]	M	43 yrs	7 days	pulmonary	CRF, depressed immunity drug	died
Sritaveesuwan and Jiamton, 1998 [13]	M	52 yrs	6 mos	cutaneous	depressed immunity drug	cured
Sitthiwong *et al.*, 2000 [11]	F	15 yrs	1 yr	subcutaneous	no data	cured
Sitthiwong *et al.*, 2000 [11]	F	27 yrs	6 mos	subcutaneous	no data	cured
Sitthiwong *et al.*, 2000 [11]	M	47 yrs	1 yr	subcutaneous	no data	cured
Krekhanjanarong and Supiyaphun, 1997 [5]	F	48 yrs	34 days	rhinocerebral	DM,CRF	no data
Krekhanjanarong and Supiyaphun, 1997 [5]	F	39 yrs	7 days	rhinocerebral	DM	no data
Krekhanjanarong and Supiyaphun, 1997 [5]	M	47 yrs	20 days	rhinocerebral	Neutropenia	no data
Krekhanjanarong and Supiyaphun, 1997 [5]	F	53 yrs	7 days	rhinocerebral	DM,CRF,HT	no data
Krekhanjanarong and Supiyaphun, 1997 [5]	F	63 yrs	30 days	rhinocerebral	DM,HT	no data
Krekhanjanarong and Supiyaphun, 1997 [5]	F	56 yrs	14 days	rhinocerebral	DM	no data
Krekhanjanarong and Supiyaphun, 1997 [5]	M	74 yrs	3 days	rhinocerebral	DM,CVA,ketoacidosis	no data
Krekhanjanarong and Supiyaphun, 1997 [5]	M	26 yrs	10 days	rhinocerebral	DM, pulmonary TB	no data

Of 27 included cases, 23 patients (85.182%) had Mucorale infection and 4 patients had Entomophthorale infection. Of these 23 patients, 52.2 % had DM, 17.4 % had CRF, 17.4 % had history of non-steroid immunosuppressive drug usage, 4.3 % had history of steroid usage and 4.3 % had prolonged antibiotic drug usage. Of 13 Mucorales-infected cases with known resulted of treatment, 9 (69.2 %) died. Concerning the left 4 patients (14.8 %) with Entomophthorales infection, all had subcutaneous zygomycosis. None of these 4 cases was died and none had underlying cause.

Concerning the duration before the admission, the patients with Mucorale visited the physician at about 20.8 days and the patients with Entomophthorale infection visited the physician at about 16.5 months.

4. DISCUSSION

In 1978, a case of mucormycosis infection in lung was noted by Piyarat [15]. This is the first report of Zygomycosis in Thailand. Then the second report of rhinocerebral mucormycosis in carvernous sinus was published by Jankun [15]. After that, there are continuously sporadic case reports in Thailand. However, there is no complete case summarization of zygomycosis in Thailand. Here, we performed a summarization on this topic.

According to our study, 27 cases in the literature were included. We detected more female cases than male zygomycosis cases. Classified into mucormycosis and entomophthoromycosis, the infections are still more common in male. Concerning the sex predominance in our series, it is not agree with the previous report that mentioned more male than female infections [8]. Concerning the patients' age, most of the patients are adults with the age range between 20 and 60 years old (21 patients, 77.8 %). This finding is also not agree with Prakitrittranon's report (1992) that showed the predominance of infection in childhood.

Classified into 5 forms of clinical manifestations of mucormycosis infection, we found that rhinocerebral mucormycosis was the most common form. In this review, as high as 59.3 % of rhinocerebral mucormycosis can be detected. This valid percentage is going in the same way as those of the previous reports, about 80% [15]. Concerning pulmonary mucormycosis, there are only 3 cases (11.1 %) in our series. This percentage is similar to that of cutaneous mucormycosis in our series. Of interest, gastrointestinal mucormycosis can be detected in only 1 case (3.7 %). Indeed, this manifestation is rare and noted in low percentage (below 7%) [1, 15]. In addition, disseminated mucormycosis, the most rare manifestation of mucormycosis [10] cannot be detected in our study. Concerning entomophthoromycosis (subcutaneous zygomycosis), there are are 4 cases or 14.8 % in this review. These cases were presented to the physician as the hard mass with clear border in subcutaneous along the arms and legs. The outside of the mass is normal, no inflammation, and no tender.

Comparing between the mucormycosis and entomophthoromycosis, the progression of the mucormycosis is more invasive and faster. In this study, the progression in the first group, took about three weeks (20.8 days) before the patient went to the hospital while the patients with entomopthromycosis wasted about one and half year before visiting the doctors (16.5 months). The patients with mycormycosis often end up with death (9/13: 69.23%), which might represent the invasiveness and the direct destruction of the tissue bringing the necrosis. Meanwhile, all patients in the entomopthromycosis group were cured to be normal. This finding may be due to the nature of entomophthoromycosis as a gradual progression with around-vessels tissue infection, not much spread, no an invasion into the lumen [8].

Concerning the underlying cause of infection, all cases with entomophthoromycosis had no cause while most of mucormycosis cases (18/23) had underlying causes. Concerning the underlying causes of mucormycosis, the most common cause is DM, which can be detected in 52.2 %. Indeed, DM and uremia bring many ketones or glucose into the blood circulation, which well serve the fungi the good environment to growth and reproduction [3]. The other underlying causes of mucomycosis are immunosuppressive and steroid drugs usage. Concerning the immunosuppressive and steroid drugs, it can inhibit the mucoral spore excretion of macrophage [3].

In conclusion, the zygomycosis in Thai patients is similar to the previous reports. However, we find a trend of female adult premodinance of infection. We also detect the trend that entomophthoromycosis shows better prognosis than mycormycosis.

5. REFERENCES

1. Abedi E, Sismanis A, Choi K, Pastore P. Twenty-five years, experience treating cerebro-orbital mucormycosis. Laryngoscope 1984; 94: 1060-2.

2. Aikvanich T, Niampradit N. Mucormycosis: a report of two cases. Thai J Dermatol 1990; 6: 113-7.

3. Chandrakul N, Sakolphadungkhet S. Mucormycosis of the cavernous sinus. Siriraj Hosp Gaz1961; 13: 327-37.

4. Cutchavaree A, Sumitsawan U, Damrongsak D, Tantachamrun T. Rhinocerebral mucormycosis (phycomycosis). J Med Assoc Thai 1978; 61: 345-51.

5. Krekhanjanarong V, Supiyaphun V. Rhinocebral mucormycosis: a 10-yea review at ChulalongKorn University Hospital. Chula Med J 1997; 41: 733-44.

6. Luxananant K. Gastric mucormycosis. Buddhachinaraj Med J 1996; 13: 131-6.

7. Nutprayun C, Kaoborisut V, Sukontaman P. Lung infiltration with hemorrhagic pleural effusion in S.L.E. Chula Med J 1979; 23: 373-91.

8. Prakitrittranon W. Subcutaneous zygomycosis(Basidiobolomycosis). Thai J Dermatol 1992; 8: 215-20.

9. Ponglertnapagorn P, Subhannachart P, Tangthangtham A, Koanantakool T. Pulmonary zygomycosis. Thai J Tuberc Chest Dis 1994; 15: 201-10.

10. Puangpornsri P, Prakitlittanon W, Eauananta Y. Mucormycosis: one case report. Khon Kaen Med J 1987; 11: 39-42.

11. Sitthiwong W, Mahaisavariya P, Chaiprasert A, Manonukul J. Chronic subcutaneous zygomycosis: three cases of entomophthoromycosis basidiobolae. Thai J Dermatol 2000; 15: 154-61.

12. Srisukwattana C, Churoj A, Tungbumpensuntorn S, Aumawat K, Sukrungraung S. Pathogenic fungi and fungal diseases. Sarnmolchon 1986: 121-7,212-4.

13. Sritaveesuwan R, Jiamton S. Mucormycosis. Thai J Dermatol 1998; 13: 217-19

14. Supasin A, Supaporn T. Infectional complication in lung after renal transplantation: report of 3 patients after renal transplantation. J Nephrol Soc Thai 1999; 4: 232-37.

15. Watcharaprechasakun V. Clinico-pathological conference III. Reg 7 Med J 1994; 13: 421-23.

16. Wiriyasatiankun S, Komolsuradej V. Mucormycosis: two cases of cerebro-rhino-orbital mucormycosis. Thai J Ophthalmol 1992; 6: 45-52.

17. Khemnak N, Ngamrassamiwong S, Wiwanitkit V. Mucorales infection as a complication of diabetes mellitus-a summary of Thai cases. Diabetologia Croatica 2005; 34: 97-9.

CHAPTER 12

NEW RESEARCHES ON MOLECULAR BIOLOGY ASPECT OF HEPATITIS VIRUS: SOME NEW EXAMPLES

Viroj Wiwanitkit[1]

[1]Wiwanitkit House, Bangkhae, Bangkok Thailand 10160

Address correspondence to: Professor Viroj Wiwanitkit, Wiwanitkit House, Bangkhae, Bangkok Thailand 10160 Email: wviroj@yahoo.com

Abstract: Hepatitis virus infection is an important infection in medicine. There are many hepatitis viruses. There are many new researches on molecular biology aspect of hepatitis viruses. The author hereby presents some new example on epitope preference in wild and mutated precore of hepatitis B virus, weak linkage in HGV 5' non-coding region and transmembrane topology of hepatitis B envelope proteins.

Keywords: hepatitis B, mutation, precore, envelop proteins, tranmembrane, topology, hepatitis G, structure, weak linkage, mutation.

1. DIFFERENCE IN EPITOPE PREFERENCE IN WILD AND MUTATED PRECORE OF HEPATITIS B VIRUS: AN EXPLANATION FOR THE PATHOGENESIS OF VACCINE ESCAPE

Introduction

Hepatitis B virus (HBV) infection is a highly contagious viral infection and can lead to chronic carrier state and the hepatocellular carcinoma in long term. Estimately 450 million people worldwide are chronically infected with HBV and are therefore at risk of developing chronic liver disorder [1]. To prevent is better than to treat of the infection. Since 1985, the number of noted and reported cases has declined as a direct result of universal immunization of neonates, vaccination of at-risk populations, lifestyle or behavioral changes in high-risk groups, refinements in the specific screening of blood donors, and the use of virally inactivated or genetically engineered products in patients with severe bleeding disorders [2]. At present, vaccination is an effective preventive measurement for this disease. HBV vaccination has effectively reduced the acute and chronic infection rates as well as other related complications in the vaccinated children [3].

Immune and antiviral selection pressures lead to vaccine or immunoglobulin escape mutants and antiviral resistant variants [3]. Precore mutant of HBV is accepted as one of the well known mutations that cause HBV vaccination escape at present [4]. Here, the author performed a bioinformatic analysis to study the change in epitope preference within the noted precore mutant of HBV comparing to the wide type.

Materials and methods

A. Getting the sequence

The database PubMed was used for searching for the amino acid sequences of wild and mutated precore of HBV. Then the derived sequences were used for further identification for epitope.

B. Prediction for T-cell epitopes by MHCPred

The author performed computation analysis to find potential T-cell epitopes for both wild and mutated precore sequences of HBV using bioinformatics tool namely MHCPred (available from the URL: http: //www.jenner.ac.uk/MHCPred) [5]. The MHCPred tool is a partial least squares-based multivariate computational statistical approach to the quantitative prediction of peptide binding to major histocompatibility complexes (MHC), the key checkpoint on the antigen presentation pathway within adaptive cellular immunity [5]. MHCPred makes use of robust statistical models for both Class I alleles (HLA-A*0101, HLAA* 0201, HLA-A*0202, HLA-

A*0203, HLA-A*0206, HLA-A*0301, HLA-A*1101, HLA-A*3301, HLA-A*6801, HLA-A*6802 and HLA-B*3501) and Class II alleles (HLA-DRB*0401, HLA-DRB*0401 and HLA-DRB*0701) (Guan *et al.*, 2003). The results of computational analysis covers peptides and their corresponding IC50 values, which implies the binding affinity. Since the previous work mentioned that HLA DRB1*0101 is an important correspondence HLA for HBV response, therefore, the author select to perform epitope prediction based on this HLA [6].

Results

- Derived sequences

According to the search, the wild and mutated precore of HBV sequences can be derived. The three studied sequences, 1 wild type and 2 mutated type are shown in Figure **1**.

1.   wild type

mqlfhlclii scscptvqas klclgwlwgm didpykefga svellsflps dffpsirdll dtasalyrea lespehcsph htalrqailc wgelmnlatw vgsnledpas relvvsylnv nmglkirqll wfhiscltfg retvleylvs fgvwirtppa yrppnapils tlpettvvrr rgrsorrrtp sprrrrsqsp rrrsqsres qc

Mutate type

2.1   AAB35291

mqlfhlclii sctcpsvqas klclgwldmd idpykefgat vellsflpsd ffpsvrdlld tasalyreal espehcsphh talrqailcw gelmtlatwv gnnledpasr dlvvnyvntn mglkirqllw fhiscltfgr etvpeylvsf gvwirtppay rppnapilst lpettvvrrr

drgrsprrrt psprrrrsqs prr

AAB35290

mqlfhlclii sctcptvqas klclgwldmd idpykefgat vellsflpsd ffpsvrdlld tasalyreal espehcsphh talrqailcw gelmtlatwv gnnledpasr dlvvnyvntn mglkirqllw fhiscltfgr etvpeylvsf gvwirtppay rppnapilst lpettvvrqr

graprrrtps prrrrsqspr r

Figure 1. Sequences of wild and mutate precore of HBV.

- Results from epitope prediction

For T-cell epitope prediction, peptides with the best predicted binding affinities for HLA DRB1*0101 in wild and mutated precores of HBV are presented in Table 1.

Table 1. Predicted binding affinities for HLA DRB1*0101 in wild and mutated precores of HBV.

	Four best predicted epitopes	**IC50value**
Wild type	155IRTPPAYRP163 58 DLLDTASAL66 47FLPSDFFPS55 104 NLEDPASRE112	1.08 1.18 1.93 1.68
Mutated type AAB35291	154IRTPPAYRP162 57 DLLDTASAL65 92ELMTLATWV100 103NLEDPASRD111	1.08 1.18 1.52 1.71
Mutated type AAB35290	154IRTPPAYRP162 57DLLDTASAL65 92 ELMTLATWV100 103 NLEDPASRD111	1.08 1.18 1.52 1.71

Discussion

In many infectious diseases, the structural aberration is believed to be the main cause of specific clinical failure in diagnosis and disease control. Some disorders are mentioned as a single substitution accompanied with other effects on the sequence frame, the others are noted as a frameshift. The mutations in HBV genes is the important cause of vaccine escape phenomenon. Of interest, the patients infected with wild type HBV initially might develop mutant strains gradually during the long course of chronic infection under the host immune pressure. Vaccine escape mutants might develop after immunoprophylaxis [7]. In addition, antiviral therapy with nucleoside analogues might also lead to drug resistant mutant strains [7]. Understanding the viral mutation status will assist to design accurate strategies of immmunoprophylaxis and antiviral therapy against HBV infection [7].

Here, the author used a computational algorithm to study the pattern of epitope preference in wild comparing to mutated type of precore HBV. Of interest, the author can identify the significant difference in best predicted epitopes among the three studied sequences. Difference in epitope binding affinities can also be demonstrated. This can be the answer that why the present HBV cannot be successful for induce the immunity in the HBV with mutated precore. In addition, the predicted epitope can be useful for further development of multiepitope vaccine to cope with the problems of precore mutate HBV.

Conclusion

HBV infection is a highly contagious viral infection and can result in chronic carrier state and the hepatocellular carcinoma in the worst case . To prevent is better than to treat of the infection. At present, vaccination is an effective preventive measurement for this disorder. Immune and antiviral selection pressures result in vaccine/immunoglobulin escape mutants and antiviral resistant variants. Here, the author performed a bioinformatic analysis to study the change in epitope preference within the noted precore mutant of HBV comparing to the wide type. For T-cell epitope prediction, peptides with the best predicted binding affinities for HLA DRB1*0101 in wild and mutated precores of HBV are predicted. The author can identify the significant difference in best predicted epitopes among the three studied sequences. Difference in epitope binding affinities can also be demonstrated. This can be the answer that why the present HBV cannot be successful for induce the immunity in the HBV with mutated precore. In addition, the predicted epitope can be useful for further development of multiepitope vaccine to cope with the problems of precore mutate HBV.

2. WEAK LINKAGE IN HGV 5' NON-CODING REGION: IDENTIFICATION OF MUTATION PRONE POINT

Introduction

Hepatitis G virus (HGV) is a specific single stranded RNA virus which represents a newly discovered virus belonging to the flavivirus family [8]. The structure of the HGV genome resembles that of HCV. HGV replicates in peripheral blood cells, while replication in liver cells has not been observed at present day [8]. Diagnosis of HGV infection is mainly by use of polymerase chain reaction (PCR), as serological techniques are still under developed [8]. Epidemiological data indicate that the virus is common throughout the world, including India and is transmitted via blood or blood products, sexually and vertically from infected mothers to children [8]. A research group at Genelabs Technologies has found out and determined the complete genomic sequence of a virus they termed HGV [9]. The genome of a newly identified virus, HGV, points to considerable homology to hepatitis C virus (HCV) [10].

Mizokami *et al.* suggested that the mutation patterns of HCV and HGV were similar to the patterns of spontaneous substitution mutations of human genes, implying that nucleotide analogue that were significantly effective against HCV and HGV might have a side effect on the normal cells of humans [11]. Presently, prediction of protein nanostructure and function is a big and interesting challenge in the proteomics and structural genomics era. To find out the point vulnerable to mutate is a new trend to expand the knowledge on disorders in genomic and proteomic level of diseases [12-13]. Generally, disordered regions in structure of a protein usually have short linear peptide motifs that are important for protein function. Identification of the peptide motifs in the amino acid sequence can give a good prediction for the weak linkages in a protein [12-13]. Here, the author performed a bioinformatic analysis to study the determine positions that trend to comply peptide motifs in the HGV 5' non-coding region.

Materials and methods

A.   Getting the sequence

The database Pubmed was used for searching for the nucleic acid sequence of HGV 5' non-coding region. Further translation of this sequence into nucleic acid sequence was performed by bioinformatics tool namely Soaplab [14]. Soaplab is a set of Web Services giving programmatic access to many applications on remote computers. Then the derived sequences were used for further study on weak linkage.

B.   Identification of weak linkage in HGV 5' non-coding region

To identify the weak linkage in HGV 5' non-coding region, a new bioinformatic tool namely GlobPlot [15] was used. GlobPlot is an example of web service that allows the user to plot the tendency within the query protein for order/globularity and disorder [15]. It successfully find out inter-domain segments having linear motifs, and also apparently ordered regions that do not contain any recognized domain [15].

LREG*DSSCACGETAHGPQVLVLPV*IRTRRQARX

Figure 1. Translational amino acid sequence of HGV 5' non-coding region.

Result

In this work, the nucleic acid sequence of isolate HGV-RT3580 5' non-coding region (AF255091) was derived from PubMed Search and was used for further study. The identified positions are presented in Figure **2**. All positions are identified as the positions resist to mutation.

lregdsscac getahgpqvl vlpvirtrrq ar

Figure 2. Identified positions (in capital) that comply peptide motifs peptide motifs in amino acid sequence of HGV 5' non-coding region.

Discussion

In many infectious disease, the structural aberration in is believed to be the main important underlying pathogenesis. Some disorders are quoted as a single substitution with other effects on the sequence frame, the others are mentioned as a frameshift. For HGV, the mutation is not well described. Mutation of hepatitis virus is an important problem leading to failure in diagnosis and treatment [16]. HGV is estimated to pose an estimated mutation rate of 3.9 x 10(-4) base substitutions per site per year [17].

Here, the author used an algorithm to identify the position in the sequence of HGV 5' non-coding region that can be mutated. According to this work, the author can identify no position. Based on this study, the weak linkages in the HGV 5' non-coding region cannot be identified and can be good information for genetic study of HGV 5' non-coding region. This can confirm a recent report that nucleotide conversions were generalized over subgenomic regions, except in the 5' untranslated region of 552 nucleotides, which was highly conserved in sequence [17]. It also imply that this region contains several blocks of highly conserved sequences that may be helpful and useful for the development of a reverse transcriptase-polymerase chain reaction (RT-PCR) assay for detection of HGV RNA [18]. In addition, the results from this study can be good data for further work on the diagnosis for mutants HGV and vaccine development.

Conclusion

Presently, prediction of protein nanostructure and function is a great challenge in the proteomics and structural genomics era. To identify the point vulnerable to mutate is a new trend to expand the knowledge on disorders in genomic and proteomic level of diseases. Here, the author performed a bioinformatic analysis to study the determine positions that trend to comply peptide motifs in the HGV 5' non-coding region. To identify the weak linkage in HDV 5' non-coding region, a new bioinformatic tool namely GlobPlot was used. According to this work, all positions are identified as the positions resist to mutation. Based on this study, the weak linkages in the HGV 5' non-coding region cannot be identified and can be good information for genetic study of HGV 5' non-coding region.

3. TRANSMEMBRANE TOPOLOGY OF HEPATITIS B ENVELOPE PROTEINS OBSERVED BY COMBINED TRANSMEMBRANE TOPOLOGY AND SIGNAL PEPTIDE PREDICTOR METHOD

Introduction

HBV particle consists of an envelope containing three related surface proteins and probably lipid and an icosahedral nucleocapsid of approximately 30 nm diameter habouring the viral DNA genome and DNA polymerase [19]. The viral envelope has three different coterminal proteins (S, M, and L proteins) spanning the membrane several times [20]. These proteins are not only expelled from viral infected cells as components of the viral envelope but in 10,000-fold excess as subviral lipoprotein particles with a diameter of 22 nm containing no capsid [20]. The three envelope proteins S, M, and L molecularly results in a complex transmembrane fold at the endoplasmic reticulum, and form disulfide-linked homo- and heterodimers [19].

Hepatitis B envelope proteins play very important role in the pathogenesis of hepatitis B. In acute HBV, immune responses relating to recovery include vigorous, polyclonal CD4 T cells directed against multiple epitopes within HBV; antibodies directed against surface envelope proteins (anti-HBs), the development of which needs the presence of a CD4 response; and HBV-specific cytotoxic T lymphocytes [21]. In addition, it is believed to be a very important factor relating to hepatitis D infection [22]. The hepatitis B envelope proteins are also present foci for vaccine and new drug search [23-25]. However, the knowledge on the structure of this protein is limited. Here, the author performed a study to determine the transmembrane region and orientation of hepatitis B envelope proteins.

Material and method

First, the sequence of the hepatitis B envelope proteins was searched from the database, PubMed. Then, the author used a tool namely Phobius for study of the transmembrane region and orientation of hepatitis B envelope proteins. Basically, this specific predictor is based on a hidden Markov model (HMM) that effectively models the different sequence regions of a signal peptide and the different regions of a transmembrane protein in a series of interconnected states [26].

Results

The sequence of hepatitis B envelope proteins is derived (BAA00944) (Figure 1). The transmembrane topology pattern is shown in Figure 2. Four transmembrane region can be seen at 63-81, 135-153, 234-256 and 263-280. Two cytoplasmic regions can be seen at 82-134 and 257-262 and the three non cytoplasmic regions can be seen at 1 -62, 154-233 and 281-281.

1 mqwnsttfhq alldprvrgl yfpaggsssg tvnpvpttas pissifsrtg dpapnmestt

61 sgflgpllvl qagfflltri ltipqsldsw wtslnflgga ptcpgqnsqs ptsnhsptsc

121 ppicpgyrwm clrrfiiflf illlclifll vlldyqgmlp vcpllpgtst tstgpcktct

181 ipaqgtsmfp sccctkpsdr nctcipipss wafarflwew asvrfswlnl lvpfvqwfag

241 lsptvwlsvi wmmwywgpsl ynilspflpl lpiffclwvy i

Figure 1. Sequences of hepatitis B envelope proteins.

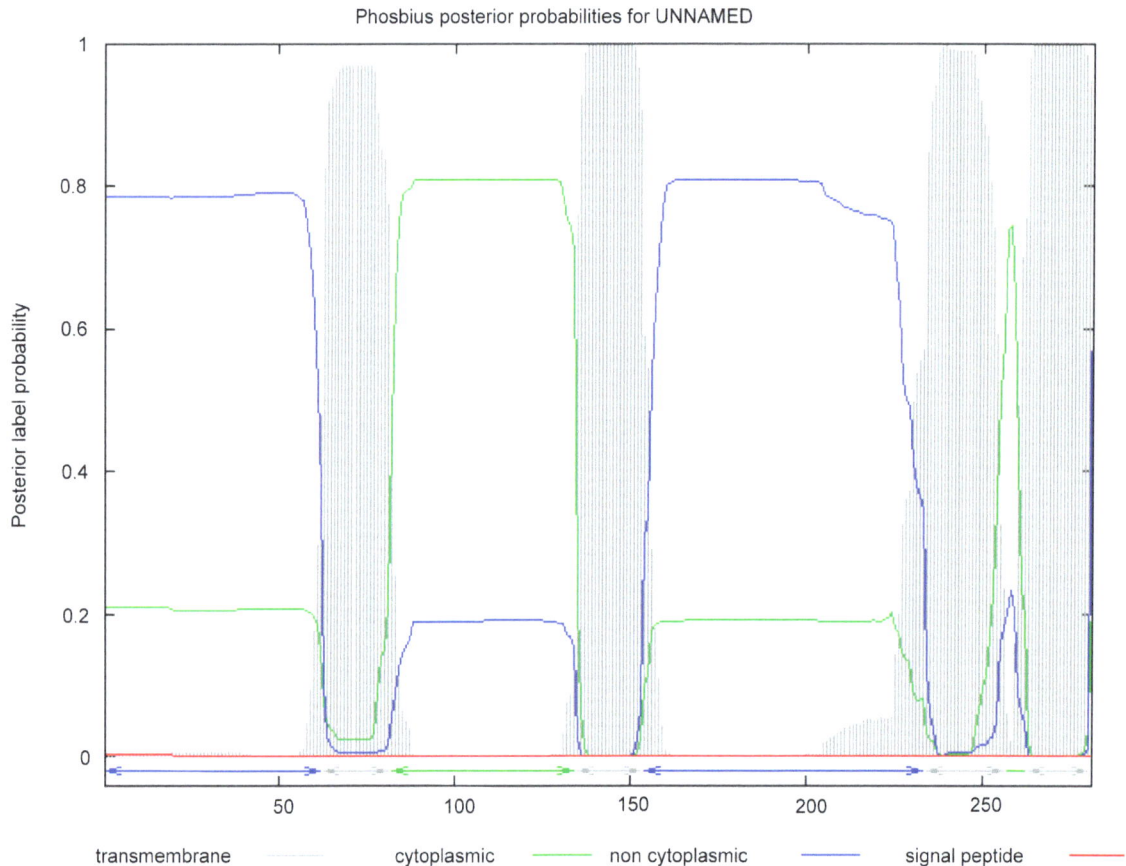

Figure 2. The transmembrane topology pattern of hepatitis B envelope proteins.

Discussion

Transmembrane proteins are an important group of proteins involved in many diverse biological functions, many of which have great impact in view of medical disease mechanism and drug discovery [27]. Despite their biological importance, it has proven very difficult to solve the structures of these mentioned proteins by experimental techniques, and so there is a great amount of pressure to develop effective methods for predicting their structure [27]. Basically, the hepatitis B virus envelope and the subviral lipoprotein particles contain three viral surface proteins (L, M, and S) which are molecularly expressed from one open reading frame by the usage of three start codons and a common stop codon [27]. A receptor for HBV on liver cells has been postulated [28]. There is increasing evidence that the binding of the HBV to the target cell surface is mediated by epitopes of the proteins of the HBV envelope [28]. It is accepted that during the life cycle of HBV the large envelope protein played a pivotal role that is related to its peculiar bi-dimensional transmembrane topology [29].

In this work, the transmembrane hepatitis B envelope proteins was studied. Although there is a previous report on the transmembrane structure of hepatitis B envelope proteins, it used different techniques with lower sensitivity [30-31]. According to this work, the author used the advanced protein topology technique to study hepatitis B envelope proteins. Indeed, protein topology is accepted as the most accurate methods in computational biology [26]. According to this study, the topology pattern of hepatitis B envelope proteins is derived. Of interest, this pattern can be useful for future drug development research.

Conclusion

The hepatitis B envelope proteins are present foci for vaccine and new drug search. The three envelope proteins S, M, and L form a complex transmembrane fold at the endoplasmic reticulum, and form disulfide-linked homo- and heterodimers However, the knowledge on the protein topology is limited. Here, the author performed a study to determine the transmembrane topology of hepatitis B envelope proteins. Four transmembrane region can be seen at 63-81, 135-153, 234-256 and 263-280. Two cytoplasmic regions can be seen at 82-134 and 257-262 and the three non cytoplasmic regions can be seen at 1 -62, 154-233 and 281-281. According to this study, the topology pattern of hepatitis B envelope proteins is derived. Of interest, this pattern can be useful for future drug development.

4. REFERENCES

1. Tarantola A, Abiteboul D, Rachline A. Infection risks following accidental exposure to blood or body fluids in health care workers: a review of pathogens transmitted in published cases. Am J Infect Control 2006; 34: 367-75.

2. Hollinger FB, Lau DT. Hepatitis B: the pathway to recovery through treatment. Gastroenterol Clin North Am 2006; 35: 425-61, x.

3. Sheldon J, Rodes B, Zoulim F, Bartholomeusz A, Soriano V. Mutations affecting the replication capacity of the hepatitis B virus. J Viral Hepat 2006; 13: 427-34.

4. Hadziyannis SJ, Papatheodoridis GV, Vassilopoulos D. Precore mutant chronic hepatitis B-approach to management. MedGenMed 2003; 5: 1.

5. Guan P, Doytchinova IA, Zygouri C, Flower DR. MHCPred: bringing a quantitative dimension to the online prediction of MHC binding. Appl Bioinformatics 2003; 2: 63-

6. Godkin A, Davenport M, Hill AV. Molecular analysis of HLA class II associations with hepatitis B virus clearance and vaccine nonresponsiveness. Hepatology 2005; 41: 1383-90.

7. Chang MH. Hepatitis B virus mutation in children. Indian J Pediatr 2006; 73: 803-7.

8. Sehgal R, Sharma A. Hepatitis G virus (HGV): current perspectives. Indian J Pathol Microbiol 2002; 45: 123-8.

9. Waqar AB, Khan S, Idrees M. Novelity in GB virus C/hepatitis G virus and its controversy. J Ayub Med Coll Abbottabad 2002; 14: 31-5.

10. Belyaev AS, Chong S, Novikov A, Kongpachith A, Masiarz FR, Lim M, Kim JP. Hepatitis G virus encodes protease activities which can effect processing of the virus putative nonstructural proteins. J Virol. 1998; 72: 868-72.

11. Mizokami M, Imanishi T, Ikeo K, Suzuki Y, Orito E, Kumada T, Ueda R, Iino S, Nakano T. Mutation patterns for two flaviviruses: hepatitis C virus and GB virus C/hepatitis G virus. FEBS Lett. 1999; 450: 294-8

12. Lee C, Wang Q. Bioinformatics analysis of alternative splicing. Brief Bioinform 2005; 6: 23-33.

13. Levin JM, Penland RC, Stamps AT, Cho CR. Using in silico biology to facilitate drug development. Novartis Found Symp 2002; 247: 222-38.

14. Senger M, Rice P, Oinn T. Soaplab-a unified Sesame door to analysis tools. Cox SJ. Proceedings, UK e-Science, All Hands Meeting 2003 2003; 509-513.

15. Linding R, Russell RB, Neduva V, Gibson TJ. GlobPlot: Exploring protein sequences for globularity and disorder. Nucleic Acids Res 2003 ; 31: 3701-8.

16. Koff RS. Problem hepatitis viruses: the mutants. Am J Med 1994; 96: 52S-56S.

17. Nakao H, Okamoto H, Fukuda M, Tsuda F, Mitsui T, Masuko K, Iizuka H, Miyakawa Y, Mayumi M. Mutation rate of GB virus C/hepatitis G virus over the entire genome and in subgenomic regions. Virology. 1997; 233: 43-50.

18. Linnen JM, Fung K, Fry KE, Mizokami M, Ohba K, Wages JM Jr, Zhang-Keck ZY, Song K, Kim JP. Sequence variation and phylogenetic analysis of the 5' terminus of hepatitis G virus. J Viral Hepat. 1997; 4: 293-302.

19. Bruss V. Hepatitis B virus morphogenesis. World J Gastroenterol 2007 Jan 7; 13(1): 65-73.

20. Bruss V. Envelopment of the hepatitis B virus nucleocapsid. Virus Res 2004 Dec; 106(2): 199-209.

21. Koziel MJ. The immunopathogenesis of HBV infection. Antivir Ther 1998; 3(Suppl 3): 13-24.

22. Taylor JM. Replication of human hepatitis delta virus: recent developments. Trends Microbiol 2003 Apr; 11(4): 185-90.

23. Shouval D. Hepatitis B vaccines. J Hepatol 2003; 39 Suppl 1: S70-6.

24. Wen YM, Lin X, Ma ZM. Exploiting new potential targets for anti-hepatitis B virus drugs. Curr Drug Targets Infect Disord 2003 Sep; 3(3): 241-6.

25. Hurwitz N, Pellegrini-Calace M, Jones DT. Towards genome-scale structure prediction for transmembrane proteins. Philos Trans R Soc Lond B Biol Sci 2006; 361: 465-75.

26. Punta M, Forrest LR, Bigelow H, Kernytsky A, Liu J, Rost B. Membrane protein prediction methods. Methods 2007; 41: 460-74.

27. Bruss V, Gerhardt E, Vieluf K, Wunderlich G. Functions of the large hepatitis B virus surface protein in viral particle morphogenesis. Intervirology 1996; 39(1-2): 23-31.

28. Theilmann L, Goeser T. Interactions of hepatitis B virus with hepatocytes: mechanism and clinical relevance. Hepatogastroenterology 1991 Feb; 38(1): 10-3.

29. Lambert C, Prange R. Development and characterization of a 293 cell line with regulatable expression of the hepatitis B virus large envelope protein. J Virol Methods 2004 Nov; 121(2): 181-90.

30. Bruss V, Lu X, Thomssen R, Gerlich WH. Post-translational alterations in transmembrane topology of the hepatitis B virus large envelope protein. EMBO J 1994 May 15; 13(10): 2273-9.

31. Prange R, Streeck RE. Novel transmembrane topology of the hepatitis B virus envelope proteins. EMBO J 1995 Jan 16; 14(2): 247-56.

INDEX